THE HERO
WORKOUTS

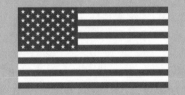

100 WORKOUTS
DEDICATED TO FALLEN
SOLDIERS & WARRIORS

RESEARCHED AND WRITTEN BY
Carter Henry

FOREWORD BY
Stewart Smith, USN (SEAL)

Hatherleigh Press is committed to preserving and protecting the natural resources of the earth. Environmentally responsible and sustainable practices are embraced within the company's mission statement.

Visit us at www.hatherleighpress.com and register online for free offers, discounts, special events, and more.

THE HERO WORKOUTS

Library of Congress Cataloging-in-Publication Data is available.

ISBN: 978-1-57826-658-6

BOOK DESIGN BY CAROLYN KASPER

The views expressed are those of the author and do not reflect the official policy or position of the US Navy, Department of Defense, or the US Government.

DEDICATION

To every Sailor, Marine, Airman, Soldier, and patriot I have had the honor of serving alongside—thank you.

SPECIAL THANKS

To my family, for their enthusiasm, support, and boundless patience; to Cherie and Stephanie, for being magnificent human beings and steadfast friends; to Erin, for always encouraging me to take the rudder; to the Curmudgeon Club, for howling down mediocrity with morose glee at every opportunity; and in memory of AGC "Libbet" Miller, who became a Navy Chief when it was still unladylike to do so.

CONTENTS

FOREWORD

The Hero Workouts is one of the most meaningful fitness books I have ever had the pleasure of reading. The workouts are great, but the story behind the workout motivates you to work hard so these heroes are never forgotten.

In the tactical profession, fitness is an element that requires your focus and time to better help you save lives—maybe even your own. Remember each of the brave heroes in this book, as well as those we could not honor due to space, as you perform any of these workouts.

It is an honor to be a part of this book in any way.

—Stew Smith
  Navy SEAL, Tactical Fitness Author

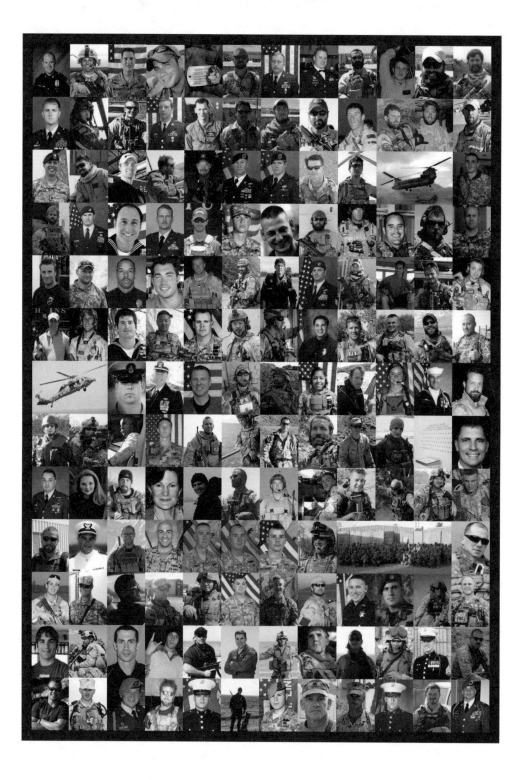

INTRODUCTION

As we express our gratitude, we must never forget that the highest appreciation is not to utter words but to live by them.

John F. Kennedy

I n 2014, I was introduced to "Hero WODs" (meaning "workout of the day")—high-intensity CrossFit workouts dedicated to those who have given their lives in service: military members, federal agents, and first responders. These memorials required more resolve than anything else I had tried before but, no matter how hard they were or how tired I felt, I pressed on, knowing that quitting was completely unacceptable. I loved what the workouts stood for, and committed myself to completing 52 Hero WODs in a year. A few months in, I realized that finishing a workout didn't have a positive impact on anyone but me, and I wanted to find a way to give back. *The Hero Workouts* is the result of what started as a personal challenge: a compendium of 100 workouts with biographies and stories about the fallen men and women whose memories they honor.

In writing and learning about these service members, I've also become more familiar with the issues faced by wounded veterans and their families. I started volunteering with another veteran aid group, believing that our Airmen, Sailors, Soldiers, and Marines deserve the support of the people they have risked their lives protecting. It has never seemed right to me that a person who has willingly committed their life to our country could be left with so little afterwards. This book has become my way of not only showing them my gratitude, but *living* it. All profits I am entitled to as the author are donated to the Special Operations Warrior Foundation to help the families of the fallen. There are many, many more workouts that have been dedicated to our national heroes, and I plan to continue publishing these workouts to raise funds for military charities.

While reading *The Hero Workouts*, you will find charitable causes associated with the honorees and their workouts. There are foundations started in their names, scholarships given in their honor, and projects to preserve their legacy, each representing the person they were, or something they believed.

So I charge you: attack these workouts. Read about the person you are honoring, and give them your greatest effort. Consider making a contribution to a charity in their name. Many of the organizations and events can benefit not only from your monetary gifts but also from donations of your time.

These heroes and their families have given more than most of us can fully appreciate, and for that they have my utmost thanks. Remember also the men and women who continue to defend our country, at home and abroad—they make us strong and will not be forgotten.

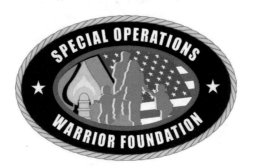

The Special Operations Warrior Foundation (SOWF) was established in 1980 after the daring attempt to rescue 53 American hostages in Iran, which ended in tragedy when a helicopter and C-130 aircraft collided; eight souls were lost and they left behind 17 children. A battlefield promise to take care of those children has become the noble cause of the SOWF.

The SOWF is committed to providing scholarship grants—not loans—to over 1,100 children, who survive more than 900 Special Operations personnel who gave their lives in service to our country. Today, the foundation ensures full financial assistance for a post-secondary degree from an accredited two- or four-year college, university, technical school, or trade school to the surviving children of Army, Navy, Air Force, and Marine Corps special operations personnel who lose their lives in the line of duty. The SOWF also provides family and educational counseling, and immediate financial assistance to severely wounded and hospitalized special operations personnel. From the date of a family's loss and for years after, the foundation maintains constant contact and offers both family and educational counseling.

In 2014, the SOWF supported 143 students enrolled across the country, and provided $3.8 million in scholarships and support services. Fifteen percent of the sale price of this book will go directly to the foundation, and will help their ongoing efforts to aid the families of fallen and injured service members. To make an additional contribution or to learn about fundraising events in your area, please visit their website at www.SpecialOps.org.

A NOTE FOR
THE WORKOUTS

The weights listed with the workouts are the "prescription" and when there are two weights shown, for example 155/125lbs, it's intended to differentiate between men/women. Using less (or more) weight doesn't degrade the integrity of the workout: it's about your personal capability and using maximum effort. If you aren't exerting yourself, add more weight; if your form is failing, use less weight. Test out the movements before starting to get a feel for where you are, and avoid having to make changes while on the clock.

Most of the weights are listed in pounds, but several of the kettlebells workouts have denominations in poods. For the equivalent in pounds, multiply the number of poods by 36.1.

THE HERO
WORKOUTS

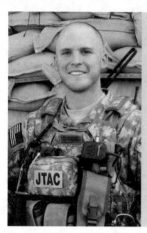

SENIOR AIRMAN BRADLEY SMITH
January 3, 2010

Photo Credit: af.mil

Brad was raised in Troy, Illinois, and followed his older brother into military service in 2006. He trained in the Air Force to direct aircraft for combat operations and qualified as a Joint Terminal Attack Controller (JTAC). In December 2009, Brad was sent to the Kandahar province of Afghanistan.

His element was on patrol they came under attack in early January, and the blast of an improvised explosive device injured three men. Along with Army medic Specialist Brian Bowman, Brad ran to recover the two casualties; he proceeded to returned fire to the enemy while coordinating three attack helicopter formations. Brad and Brian then waded into a creek to retrieve the body of the third solider. On January 3, 2010, Senior Airman Bradley Smith, 24, was killed instantly when a second IED detonated. He is survived by his widow, Tiffany; their daughter, Chloe; his parents, Gary and Paula; and his brother, Ryan. In September 2012, Brad was posthumously awarded the Silver Star for his gallantry in action and devotion to duty.

More than 30 members of Brad's squadron marched from his gravesite in Glen Carbon, Illinois to their home base in Fort Riley, Kansas—over 470 miles. Taking two-man shifts of 12 miles, they carried Brad's uniform and a memorial stone that was later placed at Fort Riley's Victory Park. Today, the Bradley R. Smith Memorial Scholarship fund carries on Brad's legacy, raising tuition money through donations and an annual 5k race. To make a donation or register for the race, visit www.RunForBrad.org.

BRADLEY

10 rounds for time:
SPRINT (100M)
10 PULL-UPS
SPRINT (100M)
10 BURPEES
[Rest 30 seconds]

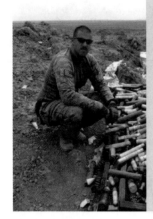

SENIOR AIRMAN BRYAN BELL

January 5, 2012

Photo Credit: C   srossfit

Bryan was a native of Eerie, Pennsylvania. He enlisted in the Air Force after graduating from Harbor Creek High School, and qualified as an Explosive Ordnance Disposal technician in 2008. While stationed with the 2nd Civil Engineer Squadron at Barksdale AFB in Louisiana, Bryan was sent to Iraq to support Operation Iraqi Freedom and, later, Afghanistan for Operation Enduring Freedom. He worked to clear supply routes, disarm ordnance, and train local forces in EOD techniques.

During his last call home, Bryan was proud to tell his father about an improvised explosive device that his unit had rendered safe. His family knew Bryan became an EOD technician because he wanted to save people, and had found his purpose in his work. On January 5, 2012, Senior Airman Bryan Bell, 23, and two other Airmen were killed when their vehicle hit an IED. He is survived by his widow, Alaina; his mother and stepfather, Brenda and David Aldrich; his father and stepmother, Richard and Kim Bell; his sister, Candace, and his stepsiblings, Stephanie and Matthew. For his sacrifice, Bryan was posthumously decorated with the Bronze Star with Valor and the Purple Heart.

If you would like to make a donation in Bryan's name, please consider the EOD Warrior Foundation, an organization committed to serving the EOD community by providing assistance and financial support in times of need. To learn more, please visit www.EODWarriorFoundation.org/Memorial/Warrior/Bryan-R-Bell.

BELL

3 rounds for time:

21 DEADLIFTS (185lbs)

15 PULL-UPS

9 FRONT SQUATS (185lbs)

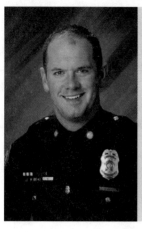

OFFICER DAVID MOORE
January 26, 2011

Photo Credit: Indianapolis Metropolitan PD

Growing up in Indianapolis, David planned to become an officer in the Marine Corps. He attended Purdue University as a midshipman in the ROTC program, but was told that an old knee injury would prevent him from commissioning. With parents who both served as police officers, David decided to pursue a career in law enforcement. He earned his degree in criminal justice and joined the Indianapolis Metropolitan Police Department in 2004. David quickly distinguished himself on the force: he was recognized in 2005 as the Rookie Officer of the Year and, in 2008, was decorated with Medal of Valor for action taken in the line of duty.

On January 23, 2011, David was performing a routine vehicle stop when the driver shot him four times before fleeing the scene. Two days later, the wounds inflicted on Officer David Moore, 29, were pronounced fatal and he was removed from life support the next morning. David is survived by his parents, Spencer and Jo; and his sister, Carol. Thomas Hardy, the man who shot David, pleaded guilty to murder and was sentenced to life in prison without parole.

Today, the Officer David S. Moore Foundation continues David's legacy of service by providing funding to community improvement initiatives. To learn more about their current projects, please visit www.DavidSMooreFoundation.org. Purdue University also established the David S. Moore Navy ROTC Scholarship for midshipmen students; additional information can be found at www.Purdue.edu/UDO/ DavidMoore.

MOORE

In 20 minutes, as many rounds as possible:

1 ROPE CLIMB (15')

RUN (400M)

MAXIMUM REPS OF HANDSTAND PUSH-UPS

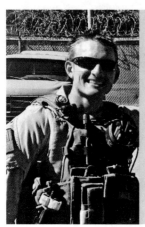

PETTY OFFICER SECOND CLASS TAYLOR GALLANT
January 26, 2012

Photo Credit: Epdwarriorfoundation.org

Taylor enlisted in the Navy in 2009, shortly after graduating from George Rogers Clark High School in Winchester, Kentucky. He was selected for the Explosive Ordnance Disposal program and, after finishing boot camp, went to Florida to attend diver training and earn his EOD qualifications. After months spent completing advanced courses like jump school and tactical combats skills instruction, Taylor reported to EOD Mobile Unit TWELVE in Virginia Beach.

On January 26, 2012, Taylor's unit was preparing to take part in an amphibious exercise off the coast of North Carolina. Petty Officer Second Class Taylor Gallant, 22, was diving from the Canadian ship HMCS Summerside (MM-711) when a training accident claimed his life. He is survived by his sons, Ethan and Harrison; their mother, Christie; his brother, Kyle; his mother, Beth; and his father, Joseph.

As the funeral procession for Taylor passed through his hometown of Winchester, hundreds of residents stood in the rain to pay their respects; many held American flags. Taylor's leadership spoke at his funeral, where they recounted his willingness to help others and his dedication to duty, his adventuring spirit and sharp intelligence.

The EOD Warrior Foundation provides support and financial assistance to EOD service members and their families. To make a donation in Taylor's honor, please visit www.EOD WarriorFoundation.org/Memorial/Warrior/Taylor-J-Gallant. Taylor is also remembered at the Patriots Peace Memorial in Louisville, Kentucky (see www.PatriotsPeaceMemorial.org).

GALLANT

For time:

RUN (1600M)*

60 BURPEE PULL-UPS

RUN (800M)*

30 BURPEE PULL-UPS

RUN (400M)*

15 BURPEE PULL-UPS

Workout Notes
*With a 20lbs medicine ball

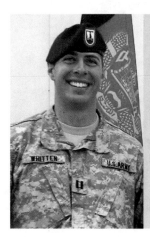

CAPTAIN DANIEL WHITTEN
February 2, 2010

Photo Credit: Crossfit

Dan graduated from Johnston High School near his hometown of Grimes, Iowa. He was selected to attend the United States Military Academy at West Point, and double-majored in English and mathematics before commissioning in the Army in 2004. The following year, just six days after his wedding, Dan left for his first deployment to Iraq. He then completed a tour of duty in Afghanistan in 2008, and returned in 2009. During his third and final deployment, Dan served as the company commander for 120 paratroopers from 1st Battalion, 508th Parachute Infantry Regiment. He loved his job, and excelled at leading his Soldiers in the austere conditions of Afghanistan.

On February 2, 2010, Dan and his men were returning from a three-day operation when their Humvee was struck by the blast of an improvised explosive device; Dan, uninjured, moved to another vehicle and the convoy pressed on. Several miles later, the detonation of another IED took the life of Captain Daniel Whitten, 28, and that of another Soldier in his company. He is survived by his widow, Starr; his mother, Jill; his father and stepmother, Dan and Penny; and his sister, Sarah. Dan was interred at West Point Cemetery, and was posthumously decorated with the Bronze Star and the Purple Heart medals in recognition of his service.

The Strong Gray Line is an anthology commemorating fallen Soldiers from the West Point Class of 2004. Created by the graduating class, the compilation supports a number of charitable causes. To learn more or to order a copy, please visit www.TheStrongGrayLine.com.

WHITTEN

5 rounds for time:

22 KB SWINGS (2 pood)

22 BOX JUMPS (24")

RUN (400M)

22 BURPEES

22 WALL BALL SHOTS (20lbs)

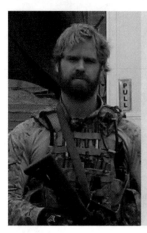

CHIEF PETTY OFFICER NATHAN HARDY
February 4, 2008

Photo Credit: Veterantributes.org

Nate graduated from Oyster River High School in Durham, New Hampshire in 1997 and left for boot camp just a few months later. After finishing Basic Underwater Demolition/SEAL training in 1999, Nate spent eight years serving with SEAL Team EIGHT in Virginia Beach and Naval Special Warfare Unit TWO in Stuttgart, Germany. He was then selected for assignment to the elite Naval Special Warfare Development Group.

Nate completed multiple tours of duty overseas in Afghanistan, Kosovo, and Iraq. During a night-time mission in Iraq on February 4, 2008, he and a teammate made entry into a building held by insurgents and were immediately struck by small arms fire. Chief Petty Officer Nathan Hardy, 29, was mortally wounded but continued to engage the enemy while dragging Chief Petty Officer Michael Koch to safety. Both men succumbed to their wounds; they are interred side-by-side in Arlington National Cemetery, section 60, stones 8567 and 8568. Nate is survived by his widow, Mindi; his son, Parker; his brother, Ben; and his parents, Stephen and Donna. For his bravery, he was posthumously awarded the Bronze Star with Valor and the Purple Heart medals.

The Bobcat Bolt is held annually in Nate's hometown to raise money for scholarship awards honoring Nate and his older brother Josh, who died of brain cancer in 1993. To register for the race, please visit www.BobCat Bolt.com. Seacoast United Soccer Club also hosts an annual soccer tournament in remembrance of Nate, and maintains the Nate Hardy International Scholarship. For more information, please visit www.SeaCoastUnited.com.

NATE

In 20 minutes, as many rounds as possible:

2 MUSCLE-UPS

4 HANDSTAND PUSH-UPS

8 KB SWINGS (2 pood)

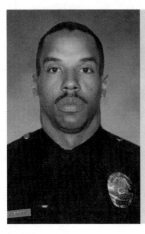

OFFICER RANDAL SIMMONS

February 7, 2008

Photo Credit: Los Angeles PD

Randy was the son of a minister, and was raised with a faith that stayed with him throughout his life. At Washington State University, he pursued his criminology degree and played cornerback on the school's football team. Randy was on the brink of becoming a professional athlete when an injury took him off the field; he then chose to attend the Los Angeles Police Academy and graduated in 1981. Randy's Christian faith reflected in everything he did: his service was exemplary, and he had a gift for communicating with people. As a minister at Glory Christian Fellowship International Church, he founded the youth outreach program Glory Kids Ministries and served as a mentor to children in his community.

On February 7, 2008, the LAPD SWAT team made entry into a house where a man claimed to have murdered three people. Randy and another officer were shot by the suspect, who was later killed in the ensuing stand-off. Officer Randal Simmons, 51, was taken to a nearby medical center, where he died of his wounds. After 27 years of service, Randy was the first LAPD SWAT officer to be killed in the line of duty. He is survived by his widow, Lisa; his children, Matthew and Gabrielle; his parents; and his sisters. Lisa Simmons is the author of his biography, *41D: Man of Valor*.

The Randal D. Simmons Outreach Foundation continues Randy's work today, helping at-risk youth and their families through programs aimed at improving quality of life, promoting health and wellness, and providing education and financial aid. To learn more about their initiatives, please visit www.RandySimmonsSWAT.com/Foundation.

RANDY

For time:

75 POWER SNATCHES (75lbs)

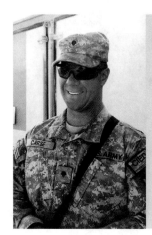

CORPORAL NATHAN CARSE

February 8, 2011

Photo Credit: Crossfit

Nathan was raised in Harrod, Ohio, and was the son of a Green Beret. He earned his undergraduate degree from Capital University before studying civil engineering and environmental science at Louisiana State University. After completing his graduate studies in 2007, Nathan was hired by a local consulting firm to help manage the reconstruction of levies in St. Bernard Parish.

In 2010, he enlisted in the Army and qualified as a combat engineer. Nathan was assigned to the 2nd Engineer Battalion, 176th Engineer Brigade at White Sands Missile Range in New Mexico and, in September of the same year, deployed to Afghanistan. On February 8, 2011, Corporal Nathan Carse, 32, was on a patrol in Kandahar province when the detonation of an improvised explosive device took his life. He is survived by his mother, Janis; his sisters, Megan and Kristin; and his girlfriend, Gerri Sanchez. In recognition of his service, Nathan was posthumously decorated with a number of awards, including the Bronze Star and the Purple Heart.

To honor his service, a portion of State Route 309 in Nathan's hometown was renamed the Army Cpl Nathan B. Carse Memorial Highway. Additionally, the Nathan Carse Memorial Scholarship is now awarded to graduating seniors at Allen East Local Schools. The scholarship fund is supported by donations and fundraisers, including an annual golf outing. Please visit the "Nathan Carse Memorial Scholarship" Facebook page for event updates and information on making a contribution in Nathan's name.

CARSE

For time, complete 21/18/15/12/9/6/3 reps in a circuit. Begin each round with a 50-meter bear crawl, then:

SQUAT CLEANS (95lbs)

DOUBLE-UNDERS

DEADLIFTS (185lbs)

BOX JUMPS (24")

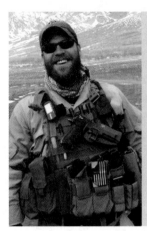

STAFF SERGEANT MARC SMALL

February 12, 2009

Photo Credit: Crossfit

Marc was raised in Collegeville, Pennsylvania and was an avid soccer player throughout high school and college. He enlisted in the Army in 2004, and began Special Forces training the following year. After earning his Green Beret and qualifying as a medical sergeant, Marc was stationed at Fort Bragg with 1st Battalion, 3rd Special Forces Group (Airborne). He deployed in January 2009 to fight insurgent forces in Afghanistan but spent much of his time providing medical care to the local population.

On February 12, 2009, Staff Sergeant Marc Small, 29, was killed during a reconnaissance patrol when enemy forces attacked his unit with rocket-propelled grenades and small arms fire. Marc is survived by his fiancée, Amanda Charney; his mother and stepfather, Mary and Peter MacFarland; his father and stepmother, Murray and Karen Small; his brother and sister, Matt and Megan; and his step-siblings, Heather, Travis, Tyler, and Jennifer.

After his deployment, Marc and Amanda had planned to open a speech therapy practice called Small Steps in Speech. Amanda, a speech pathologist, instead started a non-profit foundation by the same name to honor Marc's memory by helping children with speech and language disorders. Please visit www.SmallStepsInSpeech.org to read more about their programs. Methacton United Soccer Club also hosts the annual Marc J. Small Memorial Soccer Tournament to fund two scholarships in his name. More information can be found at www.MethactonUnited.com/MSMemorial.

SMALL

3 rounds for time:

ROW (1000M)

50 BURPEES

50 BOX JUMPS (24")

RUN (800M)

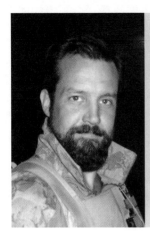

SENIOR CHIEF PETTY OFFICER THOMAS VALENTINE

February 13, 2008

Photo Credit: Arlingtoncemetery.net

Tom Valentine was a native of Ham Lake, Minnesota, where he graduated from Blaine High School. He enlisted in the Navy in 1989 and entered Basic Underwater Demolition/SEAL the following year. While assigned to SEAL Team TWO, Tom deployed overseas numerous time, including stints in the Persian Gulf, Somalia, and Kosovo. In June 1998, he successfully screened with the Navy Special Warfare Development Group and spent the remainder of his career supporting Operations Iraqi Freedom and Enduring Freedom. Throughout his life, Tom epitomized the values of the SEAL ethos: he was humble, a quiet professional with an adventurous spirit, and never gave up.

Senior Chief Petty Officer Thomas Valentine, 37, was killed in a free fall parachute training accident on February 13, 2008 in Casa Grande, Arizona; he was preparing for his tenth deployment overseas. Tom is survived by his widow, Christine; their children, John and Meghan; his parents, Jack and Katie; and his siblings, Tim and Susie. He was buried in Arlington National Cemetery in Section 60, stone 8562. During 18 years of service, Tom had been decorated with the Silver Star and three Bronze Stars with Valor.

The All In, All the Time Foundation was established in the wake of Tom's death, and now provides assistance to the families of fallen Naval Special Warfare service members. For more information about their work or upcoming events, please visit www.AIATT.org.

TOMMY V

For time:

21 THRUSTERS (115lbs)

12 ROPE CLIMBS (15')

15 THRUSTERS (115lbs)

9 ROPE CLIMBS (15')

9 THRUSTERS (115lbs)

6 ROPE CLIMBS (15')

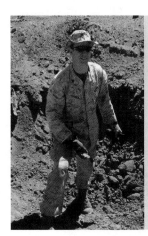

STAFF SERGEANT DANIEL HANSEN
February 14, 2009

Photo Credit: Crossfit

Daniel and his twin brother, Matthew, enlisted with the Marine Corps in 2002 after graduating from Merrill F. West High School in Tracy, California. Daniel received infantry and security forces training, and successfully screened for the presidential detail program. In May 2004, Daniel was stationed at Camp David to help guard the President and other heads of state.

A year later, Daniel was stationed with 1st Marine Division at Camp Pendleton in California and was put in charge of Major General Natonski's security detail. He was then assigned as the personal security officer for Major General Zilmer, and deployed overseas to Fallujah, Iraq in 2006. After returning to the States, Daniel took orders to Explosive Ordnance Disposal School in Florida. He completed the extensive training and was assigned to Marine Wing Support Squadron 171 in Iwakuni, Japan in 2008. Daniel was then selected for a deployment to Afghanistan.

On February 14, 2009, Sergeant Daniel Hansen, 24, was on patrol when he was killed by the detonation of a roadside bomb. He is survived by his fiancée, Emily Campbell; his parents, Delbert and Cheryll; his brother, Matthew; his sister, Katie Anne; and his half-sister, Trena. For his honorable service, Daniel was posthumously promoted to the rank of staff sergeant.

The EOD Warrior Foundation provides support and financial aid to members of the explosive ordnance disposal community and their families. To make a contribution in Daniel's name, please visit www.EOD WarriorFoundation.org/Memorial/Warrior/ Daniel-L-Hansen.

HANSEN

5 rounds for time:

30 KB SWINGS (2 pood)

30 BURPEES

30 GLUTE-HAM SIT-UPS

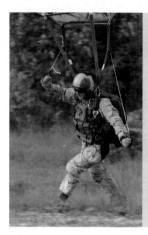

STAFF SERGEANT TIMOTHY DAVIS
February 20, 2009

Photo Credit: Crossfit

Tim grew up in Montesano, Washington. After graduating high school in 1999, he enlisted in the Air Force and worked as a survival, evasion, resistance, and escape (SERE) instructor at Fairchild Air Force Base in Washington. Tim transitioned to combat controller training in 2003 and was assigned to the 23rd Special Tactics Squadron Silver Team two years later. As a qualified Joint Terminal Attack Controller, he first deployed to Afghanistan in 2007, and volunteered to for additional duty overseas soon after returning home.

On February 20, 2009, Staff Sergeant Timothy Davis, 28, was killed when his vehicle was hit by an improvised explosive device during a combat reconnaissance patrol near Bagram. He is survived by his widow, Meagan; their son, Timmy Jr.; his mother, Sally Sheldon; his father and stepmother, Mike and Liz Davis; his siblings, Ben and Noel; and his uncle, Jim Sheldon. Tim, remembered by his commander as "the epitome of the quiet professional", was posthumously awarded the Bronze Star with Valor and the Purple Heart.

That October, 12 men left Lackland Air Force Base in Texas to complete an 800-mile memorial march in Tim's honor. Upon their arrival at Hurlburt Field in Florida, Tim's name was added to the Combat Control Memorial. The march benefited the Special Operations Warrior Foundation by raising scholarship funds for SOWF beneficiaries, and is now held every year that a Special Tactics Airman is lost. To make a donation in Tim's name, please go to www.SpecialOps.org.

DT

5 rounds for time:

12 DEADLIFTS (155lbs)

9 HANG POWER CLEANS (155lbs)

6 PUSH JERKS (155lbs)

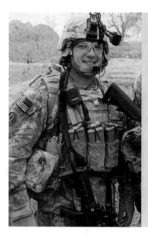

FIRST LIEUTENANT DAREN HIDALGO

February 20, 2011

Photo Credit: Crossfit

Daren was raised in Pennsylvania and came from a tradition of military service. He graduated from Dallastown Area High School in 2005 and joined his older brother at the United States Military Academy at West Point. After completing his degree in Spanish, Darren commissioned as an infantry officer in the Army. He reported to Fort Benning, Georgia to attend the Basic Airborne Course and Range School, and subsequently assigned to serve as a platoon leader with 2nd Stryker Calvary Regiment in Germany.

While deployed to the Kandahar province of Afghanistan, Daren was injured by shrapnel from an explosion and was told to have surgery. He refused, choosing instead to stay with his Soldiers. Sixteen days later, on February 20, 2011, First Lieutenant Daren Hidalgo was killed in action when his unit was hit by the blast of an improvised explosive device. He is survived by his parents, Jorge and Andrea; and his siblings, Jared, Miles, and Carmen. Daren was interred at West Point on what would have been his twenty-fifth birthday; he was laid to rest next to his friend, First Lieutenant Dimitri del Castillo, whose story can be found on page 100.

Knowing he might not return from deployment, Daren told his father that he wanted to leave a legacy of helping wounded Soldiers and supporting wrestlers from his high school. The memorial fund established in Daren's honor supports both of these causes through fundraising events and donations; to learn more, please visit www.RememberDaren.com.

HIDALGO

For time:

RUN (2 MILES)

[Rest 2 minutes]

20 SQUAT CLEANS (135lbs)

20 BOX JUMPS (24")

20 WALKING LUNGE STEPS*

20 BOX JUMPS (24")

20 SQUAT CLEANS (135lbs)

[Rest 2 minutes]

RUN (2 MILES)

Workout Notes
*Perform with a 45-lb plate held overhead

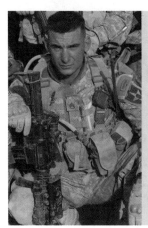

STAFF SERGEANT JOSHUA HAGER
February 23, 2007

Photo Credit: Crossfit

Josh was raised by his mother in Broomfield, Colorado and graduated from Colorado High School in 1995. He enlisted in the Army three years later and, following basic training, completed the Basic Airborne Course. Josh was first assigned to the 82nd Airborne Division at Fort Bragg and served an assignment overseas in Korea. After returning to the States, he finished Ranger School and was stationed at Eglin Air Force Base; there, Josh spent two and a half years as an instructor at the 6th Ranger Training Battalion. His next assignment was back in Colorado, at Fort Carson with 1st Battalion, 9th Infantry Regiment, 2nd Brigade Combat Team, 2nd Infantry Division.

Joshua deployed with 1st Battalion to Iraq in October 2006, and was selected for the role of Scout Platoon Sergeant. On the night of February 22, 2007, he was working as the element leader during a vehicle movement in Ramadi. Staff Sergeant Joshua Hager, 29, was killed by the detonation of an improvised explosive device. He is survived by his widow, Heather; their son, Bayley; his mother, Lois Knight; his father, Kris Hager; and his stepbrother, Aaron Jozsef. In recognition of his service, Josh was posthumously awarded the Bronze Star and the Purple Heart medals.

The Lead the Way Fund is dedicated to helping disabled Army Rangers and the families of Rangers who have died, been injured, or are currently serving in harm's way. To make a donation in honor of Josh, please visit www.LeadTheWayFund.org.

JOSH

For time:

21 OVERHEAD SQUATS (95lbs)

42 PULL-UPS

15 OVERHEAD SQUATS (95lbs)

30 PULL-UPS

9 OVERHEAD SQUATS (95lbs)

18 PULL-UPS

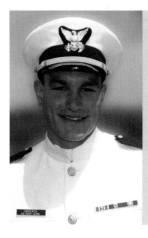

LIEUTENANT JUNIOR GRADE THOMAS CAMERON

February 28, 2012

Photo Credit: Crossfit

Tom was a lot of things: he was a fierce competitor, a loyal friend, a natural leader, and a die-hard Oregon Ducks fan. After graduating from Cleveland High School in Portland, Oregon, he was selected to attend the U.S. Coast Guard Academy. Tom played varsity soccer while majoring in Operations Research, and was awarded a spot in the Coast Guard's flight program his senior year. He commissioned as an officer following his graduation in 2009, and began primary flight training in Florida at Naval Air Station Whiting Field. Inherently dedicated to service, Tom found time to volunteer at a local correctional facility, where he helped inmates study for their GEDs.

Tom earned his gold wings and the title of Naval Aviator in 2011. He was sent to Mobile, Alabama for a final course of instruction before reporting to Coast Guard Air Station Borinquen in Puerto Rico. On February 28, 2012, Lieutenant Junior Grade Thomas Cameron, 24, was piloting a night flight when his helicopter went down in Mobile Bay; the accident claimed the lives of all four Coast Guardsmen on board. Tom is survived by his parents, John and Bette; and his brother, Alex.

At the Coast Guard Academy, Tom's jersey bears special significance; each year, one senior soccer player is selected to wear no. 12—someone who embodies Tom's legacy of leadership and hard work. Additionally, the Thomas Cameron Memorial Foundation coordinates a variety of outdoor events to benefit charity organizations and keep Tom's memory alive. To sign up for an event or learn more, please visit www.RunLiveHonor.com.

CAMERON

For time:

50 WALKING LUNGE STEPS

25 CHEST-TO-BAR PULL-UPS

50 BOX JUMPS (24")

25 TRIPLE-UNDERS

50 BACK EXTENSIONS

25 RING DIPS

50 KNEES-TO-ELBOWS

25 WALL BALL "2-FER-1"S (20lbs)

50 SIT-UPS

5 ROPE CLIMBS (15')

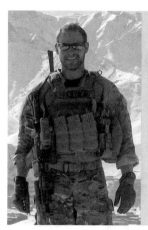

CAPTAIN ANDREW PEDERSEN-KEEL

March 11, 2013

Photo Credit: Crossfit

Andrew graduated from Avon Old Farms High School in Connecticut in 2002. Andrew commissioned in the Army as an infantry officer in 2006 and earned his Ranger tab before reporting to his first duty station in Fort Hood, Texas. In 2008, Andrew deployed to Afghanistan where, as a platoon leader, he successfully led his troops on 150 combat foot patrols and three air assault operations. He then volunteered for Special Forces and completed the Special Forces Qualification Course in 2011. Andrew was subsequently assigned to 1st Battalion, 3rd Special Forces Group as an Operational Detachment-Alpha Commander, and deployed to Afghanistan for the second time in August 2012.

Captain Andrew Pedersen-Keel, 28, was killed on March 11, 2013 when an Afghan National Policeman turned a vehicle-mounted machine gun on their Special Forces Team; Staff Sergeant Rex Schad and the team's working dog BAK were also casualties. Andrew is survived by his fiancée, Celeste Pizza; his mother and stepfather, Helen Pedersen Keiser and Bob Keiser; his father, Henry Keel; and his sister Mary Elizabeth. He was interred in Arlington National Cemetery in Section 60, stone 10108, and was posthumously awarded a third Bronze Star, the Meritorious Service Medal, and the Purple Heart.

APK Charities, a non-profit organization established in Andrew's memory, raises funds for the Connecticut Trees of Honor Memorial, the Fisher House, and the Special Forces Charitable Trust. To learn more about their upcoming events, please visit www.APKCharities.org.

PK

5 rounds for time:
10 BACK SQUATS (225lbs)
10 DEADLIFTS (275lbs)
SPRINT (400M)
[Rest 2 minutes]

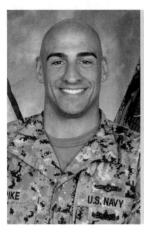

CHIEF PETTY OFFICER CHRISTIAN PIKE
March 13, 2013

Photo Credit: Goatlocker.org

Chris graduated from Peoria High School in Arizona in 2000, and enlisted in the Navy soon after. He received training as a cryptologic technician and spent the next five years aboard the USS Cleveland (LPD-7), to include multiple deployments in the Western Pacific. In 2007, Chris transferred to a unit in San Diego to support operations in the Pacific theater; he additionally volunteered for, and served, a deployment to Iraq. Chris was then selected for an assignment in Naval Special Warfare in 2011 and reported to Support Activity ONE in Coronado, California.

Chris next deployed to Afghanistan with a platoon from SEAL Team FIVE. On March 10, 2013 he warned his unit that an engagement with the enemy was imminent and badly wounded in the ensuing fight. Chief Petty Officer Christian Pike, 31, died three days later at Landstuhl Regional Medical Center in Germany. He is survived by his fiancée, Morgan Lakner; his mother, Diana; and his sister, Denise. Chris was laid to rest in Arlington National Cemetery in Section 60, stone 10553, and was posthumously awarded the Bronze Star with Valor and the Purple Heart.

In 2014, Chris' name was etched into the NSA/CSS Cryptologic Memorial Wall, joining those of 172 other men and women who have given their lives while serving in silence. To make a donation in Chris' honor, please consider the Navy SEAL Foundation, an organization that provides for Naval Special Warfare personnel and their families in times of need. Visit them at www.NavySEALFoundation.org.

PIKE

5 rounds for time:

20 THRUSTERS (75lbs)

10 RING DIPS*

20 PUSH-UPS

10 HANDSTAND PUSH-UPS*

BEAR CRAWL (50M)

Workout Notes
*Strict—no kipping

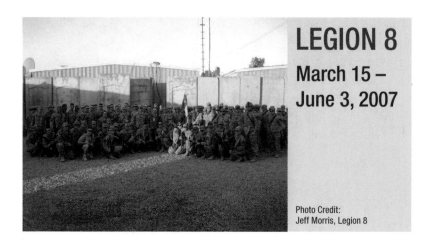

LEGION 8
March 15 – June 3, 2007

Photo Credit:
Jeff Morris, Legion 8

2007 was the deadliest year of the war in Iraq for the United States Armed Forces, and cost the lives of 904 American service members. Eight of those men were serving in Company Bravo, 1st Battalion, 8th Calvary Regiment, 2nd Brigade Combat Team, 1st Cavalry Division, based at Fort Hood in Texas. They were also simply called, "The Legion".

On March 15 of that year, their unit was on patrol when another vehicle was hit by an improvised explosive device. The Soldiers dismounted to clear the area when a second bomb detonated. Specialist Arnold, Sergeant Brand, Staff Sergeant Harris, and Staff Sergeant Prater were instantly killed; Sergeants Lightner and Green were gravely injured. Specialist Coon ran under fire to help them, applying tourniquets to stop the bleeding. In spite of surviving the evacuation, both men died of their injuries within a few days. Nearly three weeks later, Specialist Coon was shot in the head during a patrol, and Sergeant Christopher was killed in June by another IED. For their sacrifice, all eight men were awarded the Bronze Star and Purple Heart medals.

Legion 8 workout events pay tribute to these eight Soldiers, carrying on their memory and raising funds to benefit local military charities. To make a donation or to sign up for an event, please visit www.Legion8.com.

LEGION 8

8 rounds for time:

8 THRUSTERS

8 CHEST-TO-BAR PULL-UPS

8 CLAPPING PUSH-UPS

8 POWER SNATCHES

8 KNEES-TO-ELBOWS

8 SUMO DEADLIFT HIGH PULLS

8 HANDSTAND PUSH-UPS

8 TOES-TO-BAR

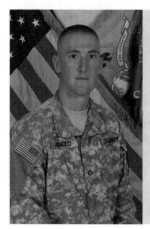

SPECIALIST JAMES ARNOLD

Photo Credit: Goldstarfamilyregistry.com

Jimmy was from Mattawan, Michigan. He played hockey at Mattawan High School, and also enjoyed playing paintball. The son of a firefighter, Jimmy was also a cadet at the Mattawan Fire Department. His work ethic and caring nature set him apart from his peers, even as a teenager. After the events of 9/11, Jimmy decided that he wanted to join the military; he enlisted in the Army in 2005 and was stationed with the 8th Cavalry Regiment at Fort Hood in Texas. Jimmy was dedicated to his brothers in uniform from the minute he entered service: he once called home to ask his mother to attend the funerals of local Soldiers as a show of support.

On March 15, 2007, Specialist James Arnold was engaged in combat operations in Iraq when he and five of his teammates were killed by the detonation of an improvised explosive device. He leaves behind his mother, Mary Ryan-Skolasky; his father, Philip Arnold; and his sisters, Amanda, Laura, Christy, and Michelle. In lieu of flowers, Jimmy's family requested memorial donations be made to the Mattawan Public Education Foundation, which awards the James Arnold Leadership Scholarship to a graduating varsity athlete who embodies Jimmy's spirit of leadership and service. To make a contribution, please visit www.MPEF.org.

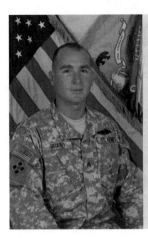

SERGEANT EMERSON BRAND

Photo Credit: Jeff Morris, Legion 8

Emerson devoted nine years of his life to the Army. After completing deployments to Kosovo and Iraq, he was selected for duty with the 3rd U.S. Infantry Regiment, the Army's official ceremonial unit in Washington D.C. "The Old Guard", as they are also known, participate in over 6,000 ceremonies a year and are responsible for standing watch at the Tomb of the Unknown Soldier. At Fort Hood, the 2nd Brigade Combat Team was scheduled for a deployment to Iraq; Emerson requested a transfer and, in 2006, relocated to Texas. He met his fiancée, Debra, soon after, and it wasn't long before he was spending his weekends with her and her children in Caddo Mills. To Emerson, who had moved frequently during his childhood, the town became the place he called "home".

Emerson returned to Iraq in 2006. When he wasn't on patrol, he was working out, preparing himself to attend the Army's Ranger course after deployment. On March 15, Sergeant Emerson Brand, 29, was one of six Soldiers killed by an improvised explosive device. His body was returned to Caddo Mills, where he received a hero's welcome home. Emerson is survived by his fiancée, Debra; and his parents, John and Debi.

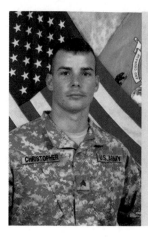

SERGEANT CALEB CHRISTOPHER

Photo Credit: Jeff Morris, Legion 8

Caleb was taking classes at Arizona State University when the terrorist attacks of September 11, 2001 took place. Born and raised in the nearby city of Chandler, he had graduated a year before in the inaugural class of Hamilton High School. Caleb left ASU to enlist in the Army, and in 2002 was assigned to the 82nd Airborne Division at Fort Bragg in North Carolina. He completed two deployments, one to Afghanistan and one to Iraq, before spending a year in California as a recruiter.

Despite the four years he spent in school as a wrestler, Caleb had a gentle nature and an uncanny knack for playing Scrabble. He enjoyed taking road trips with his fiancée and listening to music while they drove; his favorite song was "Simple Man" by Lynyrd Skynyrd.

Caleb's next assignment put him back in the infantry with the 1st Cavalry Division at Fort Hood in Texas; he left with them in October 2006 for his second tour of duty in Iraq. On June 3, 2007, Sergeant Caleb Christopher, 25, was killed when an improvised explosive device detonated near his vehicle. He leaves behind his fiancée, Rebecca Cadro; his father, Edward; and his siblings, Jeremiah, E-Jay, and Sarah. Caleb's family members all proudly wear a star tattoo in his memory.

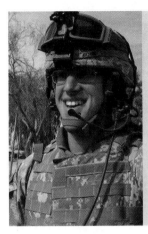

SPECIALIST JAMES COON

Photo Credit: Jeff Morris, Legion 8

James grew up near San Francisco, in the town of Walnut Creek. He attended Las Lomas High School followed by Diablo Valley College, and played football at both schools. James loved riding his motorcycle and was skilled at throwing darts; as a teenager, he represented the U.S. at an international competition in England. With his happy-go-lucky nature and outgoing personality, James made friends easily and didn't worry about much. He was also practical and knew joining the military could help him become more financially stable, and save for his own home. James enlisted in the Army in September 2005, shortly after his twenty-first birthday.

Five months into his first deployment, James saw six of his teammates hit by an IED blast. He ran to help Sergeants Green and Lightner, applying tourniquets to stop the massive bleeding. Though James bought them time, both Soldiers later died from their wounds.

On April 4, 2007, Specialist James Coon, 22, was serving as a gunner during a patrol in Balad when he was shot and killed by a sniper. He is survived by his father, Jim Coon; his half-sisters, Roxanna Coon and Samantha Lares; and his beloved dog, Tyson. James' stepmother, Marie, passed away in 2009. In lieu of flowers, his family requested donations be made in James' name to Blue Star Moms, an organization dedicated to caring for troops at home and abroad. To learn about supporting their programs, please visit www.BlueStarMoms.org.

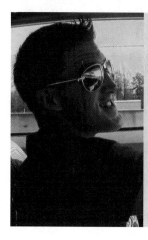

SERGEANT RYAN GREEN

Photo Credit: Jeff Morris, Legion 8

Ryan enlisted in the Army on September 12, 2001. Growing up, his family instilled in him the importance of dedication to God, country, and family; his mother wasn't surprised when, in the wake of the 9/11 terrorist attacks, Ryan showed up at home and asked for her blessing to join the military. Before that day, he had considered becoming a minister.

On March 15, 2007, Ryan was serving his second tour of duty in Iraq when he was severely injured by the detonation of an improvised explosive device. Specialist Coon applied a tourniquet to his leg, and Ryan was evacuated to a hospital where, over a series of surgeries, shrapnel was removed from his body and his leg was amputated. Sergeant Ryan Green, 24, was transported to Landstuhl, Germany for additional treatment but succumbed to his wounds on March 18, 2007. He is survived by his fiancée, Cassie Keating; his mother and stepfather, Lynda and Craig Kagan; and his step-sisters, Amanda and Jennifer Kagan. Shortly before Ryan passed away, his commanding officer presented him with the Purple Heart.

Ryan's family began the Patriot 29 Troop Support Fund to honor his memory and help support military service members. Every Independence Day, they host "Freedom Fest" at their home in Red Oak, Texas to raise money for the fund. For more information on the event or to make a donation in memory of Ryan, please e-mail Danny Roland at hooproland@yahoo.com.

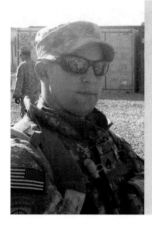

STAFF SERGEANT BLAKE HARRIS

Photo Credit: Jeff Morris, Legion 8

Blake enlisted in the Army in 1997, shortly after graduating from Lovejoy High School in Hampton, Georgia. He was initially stationed with the 82nd Airborne Division at Fort Bragg in North Carolina, and completed a tour of duty with the unit in Afghanistan. Blake's next assignment took him to Germany with the 1st Armored Division and he deployed again, this time to Iraq. After returning home, Blake transferred to the 1st Cavalry Division and relocated his family to the town of Belton, Texas.

When he deployed to Iraq again in 2006, Blake's greatest fear was that he would not be able to bring all of his men home safely. He had no fear for himself, telling his father, "…when God calls you home, you go."

On March 15, 2007, Staff Sergeant Blake Harris, 27, was killed by the detonation of an improvised explosive device. His sister-in-law, Amanda, had served with him in Germany and Iraq, and accompanied his body home to be interred at Arlington National Cemetery; Blake's final resting place can be found at Section 60, stone 8612. He is survived by his widow, Brandy; their son, Tyrus; his parents, Paul and Anne; and his siblings, Eric and Holli.

To honor Blake's memory, his family requested donations be made to Children and Adults with Attention-Deficit/ Hyperactivity Disorder, an organization dedicated to providing education, advocacy, and support for individuals with ADHD. Please visit their site at www.CHADD.org.

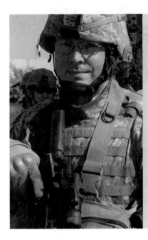

SERGEANT NICHOLAS LIGHTNER

Photo Credit: Jeff Morris, Legion 8

Nick was brought up in Newport, Oregon and graduated from Toledo High School 1996. He then spent several years working for a local distribution business and serving as a volunteer firefighter before he decided to enlist in the Army. No one was surprised when Nick began training as a combat medic, a job that would require both his physical strength and compassionate nature. In 2006, he deployed to Iraq with Company B as the platoon medic, earning the standard title of "Doc".

On March 15, 2007, Nick attempted to help Sergeant Green after he was hit by the blast of an improvised explosive device, despite being gravely injured himself. Specialist Coon rendered aid to both men, who were evacuated to receive additional medical care. Sergeant Nicholas Lightner, 29, lived for six days after the attack, but died of his wounds on March 21. For his actions on the day of the attack, he was posthumously awarded the Bronze Star, the Purple Heart, and the Combat Medical Badge. Nick is survived by his father and stepmother, Bill and Sheryl; his brothers, Josh and Nathan; his step-brothers, Justin, Alex, and Cory Lake; and his fiancée, Ginger Warfield. His story can also be found in *When It Mattered Most* by S. Ward Casscells, a memorial compilation about medical personnel killed during operations in Iraq and Afghanistan.

Nick's family requested that donations in his name be given to Fisher House, an organization that provides financial aid and support to military families during times of need. To learn more, please visit www.FisherHouse.org.

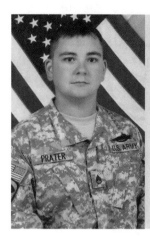

STAFF SERGEANT TERRY PRATER

Photo Credit: Jeff Morris, Legion 8

Terry grew up in Kentucky and had a deep love for the outdoors. He graduated from Powell Valley High School in Speedwell, Tennessee in 1999, and spent the next two years working in coal mines. After enlisting in the Army, Terry completed his advanced and basic training at Fort Benning, Georgia before reporting to Fort Hood, Texas.

In 2004, Terry was on his first tour of duty in Iraq when he saved the life of Sergeant Tim Ngo by shielding him from a grenade. A second blast wounded Terry; he lost part of his jawbone and his body was riddled with shrapnel. Although his injuries afforded him the opportunity to leave the military on disability, Terry fought to stay on active duty. He was later awarded the Silver Star and the Purple Heart medals for his selfless actions in defense of another Soldier.

Terry was stationed with the 1st Cavalry Division when he deployed to Iraq in October 2006. Staff Sergeant Terry Prater, 25, was killed by the detonation of an improvised explosive device on March 15, 2007. He is survived by his widow, Amy; his children, Bryson and Madisen; his mother and stepfather, Cheryl and Bruce Hurley; his father and stepmother, Terry D. and Elizabeth Prater; and his brothers, Shane Prater and Ilas Hurley. For his memorial service, friends and family gathered together at one of Terry's favorite fishing spots, Lake Norris in Tennessee, and scattered his ashes across the lake.

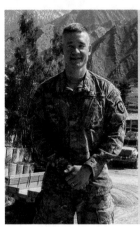

FIRST LIEUTENANT CLOVIS RAY
March 15, 2012

Photo Credit: Crossfit

Clovis was born at Fort Sam Houston in Texas, and was raised in nearby Three Rivers. He and his twin brother, Eddie, both played football at the local high school and continued to share the field at Macalester College in Saint Paul, Minnesota.

Driven by a call to serve his country, Clovis walked away from his job in investment banking at the age of 32 and commissioned in the Army in 2010. His first duty station was at Shofield Barracks, Hawaii with 2nd Battalion, 35th Infantry Regiment, 3rd Brigade Combat Team, 25th Infantry Division. Clovis deployed ahead of schedule to relieve another lieutenant who had been injured, and was scheduled to return home from Afghanistan in April 2012.

First Lieutenant Clovis Ray, 34, was mortally wounded March 15, 2012 when insurgents attacked his platoon with an IED. He was posthumously awarded the Bronze Star, Purple Heart, and NATO Medal, and was laid to rest in Arlington National Cemetery in Section 60, stone 10425. Clovis is survived by his widow, Shannon; his son, Dean; his parents, Bob Ben Sr. and Cecilia; and his siblings, Jennifer and Eddie.

In 2012, the town of Three Rivers declared that July 6th, Clovis' birthday, would be officially recognized as Clovis Ray Day from that year on. Additionally, the Clovis T. Ray Scholarship is awarded annually to a Three Rivers High School student who exemplifies the qualities that Clovis lived by: courage, leadership, and a dedication to excellence. To learn more, please visit www.Clovis RayScholarship.org.

CLOVIS

For time, and partition as needed:

RUN (10 MILES)

150 BURPEE PULL-UPS

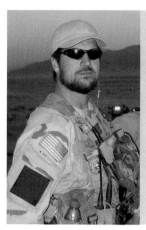

CHIEF PETTY OFFICER ADAM BROWN

March 17, 2010

Photo Credit: Adamslegacy.com

Adam was a native of Hot Springs, Arkansas. In his early twenties, Adam struggled with drugs and alcohol and began accumulating felony warrants. He was eventually arrested and given the option to spend a year in a faith-based program to help control his addiction. With the charges against him dropped and a fresh start, Adam took his life in a new direction: he got married and enlisted in the Navy. Infamous for never doing anything halfway, Adam decided to become a SEAL. He graduated from Basic Underwater Demolition/SEAL training in 2000 and served with SEAL Team FOUR and, later, Team TWO in Virginia Beach.

Adam was assigned to the Naval Special Warfare Development Group when he deployed to Afghanistan in 2010. On March 17, a number of his teammates became entrenched by heavy fire during an assault. Chief Petty Officer Adam Brown, 36, was killed in action when he charged the enemy and drew fire away from his fellow SEALs. He is survived by his widow, Kelly; their children, Nathan and Savannah; his parents, Larry and Janice; and his siblings, Shawn and Manda. For his dedication to duty, Adam was posthumously awarded the Silver Star.

Eric Blehm is the author of Adam's biography, titled *Fearless*. In his hometown, The Adam Brown 5k Shamrock Run is held annually to raise money for the Adam Brown Legacy Fund. To sign up for the race or to make a donation, please go to www.AdamsLegacy.com.

ADAM BROWN

2 rounds for time:
24 DEADLIFTS (295lbs)
24 BOX JUMPS (24")
24 WALL BALL SHOTS (20lbs)
24 BENCH PRESSES (195lbs)
24 BOX JUMPS (24")
24 WALL BALL SHOTS (20lbs)
24 CLEANS (145lbs)

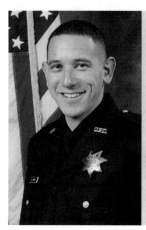

SERGEANT DANIEL SAKAI
March 21, 2009

Photo Credit: Oakland PD

After growing up in Big Bear Lake, California, moved to the Bay Area to attend the University of California, Berkeley. He completed his forestry degree in 1996, and spent a year in Japan teaching English before joining the Oakland Police Department in 2000. Daniel was initially assigned to work as a patrol officer, but served in several other roles, including academy firearms instructor and canine handler. He was promoted to Sergeant in 2007 and later became a leader of the SWAT entry team.

On March 21, 2009, Daniel's team was called to an apartment where a felon named Lovelle Mixon had barricaded himself after killing two police officers. Sergeant Daniel Sakai, 35, and another officer were fatally shot when they made entry; the remaining SWAT team members returned fire and killed the assailant. Daniel leaves behind his widow, Jennifer; their daughter, Jojiye; his parents, Tom and Mikki; and his siblings, Toshi and Tommy. The four officers killed were honored during a ceremony on March 27, and more than 20,000 people attended to pay their respects. All 815 members of the Oakland Police Department were present, with California Highway Patrol and neighboring police forces guarding the city in their absence.

The Oakland Police Foundation is dedicated to serving the police officers and at-risk youth of their city through geared toward strengthening ties between the police force and residents of Oakland. To read more about upcoming events or to make a contribution, please visit www.OaklandPoliceFoundation.org.

DANNY

In 20 minutes, as many rounds as possible:

30 BOX JUMPS (24")

20 PUSH PRESSES (115lbs)

30 PULL-UPS

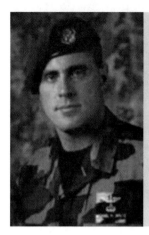

MASTER SERGEANT MICHAEL MALTZ
March 23, 2003

Photo Credit: Deamaltzchallenge.com

Mike grew up on Long Island and enlisted in the Air Force after graduating high school in 1978. He spent the beginning of his career working in communications and electronics, but later qualified for the Air Force's elite Pararescue teams. Mike went on to serve with squadrons in Florida, Alaska, Texas, and Georgia, where he jumped from planes, rescued the stranded and injured, and helped to train new PJs. He also completed multiple overseas deployments, and eventually became the poster boy of Air Force Pararescue: his picture was featured on the program's recruiting pamphlet.

While assigned to the 38th Rescue Squadron at Moody AFB, Georgia, Mike deployed to Afghanistan in 2003. On March 23, he was part of a rescue mission to help two injured children near Ghazni. Master Sergeant Michael Maltz, 42, was on board a HH-60 Pave Hawk helicopter when it crashed, taking his life and those of five other Airmen. He is survived by his sons, Kyle and Kody; his mother, Patricia Iverson; his father, John Maltz; and his siblings, Terri, Derek, and Richard.

In 2006, four DEA Special Agents started the Maltz Challenge in Mike's honor. There is no entry fee, but proceeds from the sale of memorial t-shirts benefit Homes for Our Troops, an organization dedicated to building specially adapted, mortgage-free homes for the most severely injured troops returning from the wars in Iraq and Afghanistan. To sign up for the Maltz Challenge or to make a donation in honor of Mike, please visit www.DEAMaltzChallenge.com or www.HFOTUSA.org.

FULL MALTZ

For time:

RUN (400M)

50 PULL-UPS

FIREMAN'S CARRY (100M)*

50 DIPS

100 PUSH-UPS

50 KNEES-TO-ELBOWS

100 SIT-UPS**

RUN (400M)

Workout Notes
*As an option, you may substitue Farmer's Walk
with dumbbells (200M 50/25lbs)
**Feet anchored

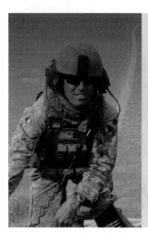

SERGEANT MAJOR ROBERT COTTLE
March 24, 2010

Photo Credit: Rickcentanni.org

Raised in Whittier, California, RJ enlisted in the Marine Corps after graduating high school in 1983. He transitioned to the reserves seven years later and joined the Los Angeles Police Department. While on the force, RJ worked assignments in Hollywood Division's vice squad and as a tactical diver. He later join the SWAT team, and served alongside Officer Randall Simmons (see page 16).

Having already served two tours in Iraq, RJ deployed to Afghanistan in 2009 with the 4th Light Armored Reconnaissance Battalion from Camp Pendleton. Sergeant Major Robert Cottle, 45, was killed during a patrol in the Helmand province on March 24, 2010 when his vehicle struck a roadside bomb; the explosion also took the life of Lance Corporal Rick Centanni. RJ is survived by his widow, Emily; their daughter, Kaila Jane; his mother, Janet Deck; his father, Kenneth Cottle; and his sister, Bonnie Roybal. He was interred at Arlington National Cemetery in Section 60, stone 8192, and was posthumously awarded the Bronze Star with Valor and the Purple Heart. RJ was the first officer from the LAPD to be killed in combat in Afghanistan.

RJ was a friend and mentor to Rick, who was only 19 years old when they were killed. The Rick Centanni Memorial Foundation hosts the annual Centanni-Cottle Memorial 5k race to honor their memories; the proceeds of the race benefit multiple charities, including the trust established by the LAPD for Emily and Kaila Jane Cottle. To make a contribution in memory of RJ, please visit www.RickCentanni.org/5k/.

RJ

5 rounds for time:
RUN (800M)
5 ROPE CLIMBS (15')
50 PUSH-UPS

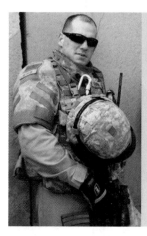

STAFF SERGEANT TRAVIS GRIFFIN
April 3, 2008

Photo Credit: Kirtland.af.mil

Travis was born in Okinawa, Japan. With his mother and stepfather both serving on active duty, he moved frequently and grew up on military bases. Travis enlisted in the Air Force in 1999 and was initially assigned to Moody Air Force Base in Georgia to serve with the 822nd Security Forces Squadron. In 2003, he transferred to Kirtland Air Force Base in New Mexico to work as a deployment trainer for the 377th Security Forces Squadron. Travis' commitment to helping others made him the ideal Airman for the job; he was funny, enthusiastic, determined, and completely dedicated to preparing Airmen for duty overseas.

In 2007, Travis volunteered for a year-long deployment with the 732th Expeditionary Security Forces Squadron —his fourth to Iraq. The Defenders in Detachment Three were working to build up the local police force and left the relative safety of base almost daily. On April 3, 2008, Staff Sergeant Travis Griffin, 28, was on patrol when an improvised explosive device detonated under his vehicle; despite the efforts of an Army medic, he succumbed to his wounds. Travis is survived by his widow, Krista; their son, Elijah; and his mother and stepfather, Christine and Donald Herwick III. In recognition of his honorable service, Travis was posthumously awarded the Bronze Star with Valor, the Purple Heart, and the Air Force Combat Action Medal.

Travis' fellow Defenders started a memorial scholarship in his name; the fund support the education goals of wounded Defenders and family members of the fallen. To make a donation, please visit www.ForGriff.com.

GRIFF

2 rounds for time:

RUN (800M)

RUN BACKWARDS (400M)

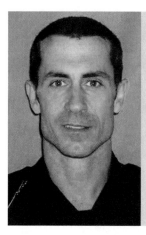

OFFICER
PAUL SCIULLO II
April 4, 2009

Photo Credit: Pittsburgh PD

Paul was raised in the Bloomfield neighborhood of Pittsburgh. He grew up playing hockey, first at the local parks, then as the captain of the team at Central Catholic High School, and later at Duquesne University. Always close to his family, Paul famously went back to his home on Pearl Street every night for dinner during college. He worked at several desk jobs after graduating, but wanted to make a difference in his community. In October 2007, Paul answered the call to serve and joined the Pittsburgh Police Department.

Officer John Sciullo, 36, was shot and killed on April 4, 2009 while answering a domestic disturbance call; Officers Stephen Mayhle and Eric Kelly were also killed, and two additional officers were injured in the ensuing shootout. The gunman, Richard Poplawski, was convicted on three counts of murder in the first degree and has remained on death row since 2011. Paul is survived by his parents, Max and Sue; and his siblings, Laura, Eric, and Julia.

On August 21, 2009, a little league field in Bloomfield was dedicated to Paul. The community landmark now bears his name and badge number, and will serve as a memorial to Paul and the sacrifice he made to the city of Pittsburgh. The Central Catholic hockey team also retired Paul's jersey, no. 20, and the school established the Paul J. Sciullo II Scholarship Fund as part of their tuition assistance program. To learn more, please visit the "Endowment" page at www.CentralCatholicHS.com.

PAUL

5 rounds for time:

50 DOUBLE-UNDERS

35 KNEES-TO-ELBOWS

OVERHEAD CARRY (20 YARDS)*

Workout Notes
*With 185lbs barbell

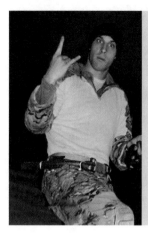

SERGEANT JASON SANTORA

April 23, 2010

Photo Credit: Crossfit

Jason grew up in the town of Farmingville on Long Island. He graduated early from Sachem North High School in 2003, and enlisted in the Army three years later. At Fort Benning, Georgia, Jason completed the Basic Airborne Course, followed by the Ranger Indoctrination Program. He was then assigned to Headquarters and Headquarters Company, 3rd Battalion, 75th Ranger Regiment, where he would serve as a mortarman and rifle team leader.

Jason returned to the Middle East in 2010 on his fourth deployment. On April 23, his platoon was hunting down a suicide attack facilitator in the Logar province of Afghanistan, and were in the process of clearing a compound when a group of civilians became stuck in the crossfire. Jason and another Ranger quickly moved into the building and up the stairs to engage the insurgents, allowing the women and children to be moved to safety. Sergeant Jason Santora, 25, was shot five times by enemy fighters and later died of his wounds; Sergeant Ronald Kubik was also killed during the mission. Both men were posthumously awarded the Silver Star. Jason was additionally decorated with the Purple Heart, Bronze Star, and the Meritorious Service Medal. He is survived by his father, Gary; and his sister, Gina. His mother, Theresa, passed away in 2013.

To make a contribution in Jason's name, please consider the Lead the Way Fund. Dedicated to Rangers and their families, the organization provides support and assistance in times of need. Please visit them at www.LeadTheWayFund.org.

SANTORA

3 rounds for reps, 1 minute per event:

SQUAT CLEANS (155lbs)

20' SHUTTLE SPRINTS*

DEADLIFTS (245lbs)

BURPEES

JERKS (155lbs)

[Rest]

Workout Notes
* 20' forward and 20' backwards equals one rep

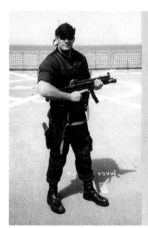

PETTY OFFICER THIRD CLASS NATHAN BRUCKENTHAL

April 24, 2004

Photo Credit: CGTLE.org

Nate was a native of Stony Brook, New York, and enlisted in the Coast Guard after graduating from Herndon High School in Virginia. He initially trained as a damage controlman, and served on the USCGC Point Wells (WPB-82343), based out of Montauk in New York. Nate then spent two years stationed in Neah Bay, Washington before accepting a position with a Tactical Law Enforcement Team based at Air Station Miami.

After completing a deployment to Iraq in 2003, Nate volunteered to return to the Middle East. He was sent to the Persian Gulf and served aboard the USS Firebolt (PC-10) as a member of the boarding team. On April 24, 2004, Petty Officer Third Class Nathan Bruckenthal, 24, died of injuries sustained when suicide bombers on board a suspicious vessel detonated their explosives. The attack took the lives of two Navy Sailors, and marked the first death of a Coast Guardsman since the Vietnam War. Nathan is survived by his widow, Pattie; his mother, Laurie Bullock; his father Ric Bruckenthal; and his siblings, Noabeth, Matthew, and Michael. His daughter, Harper, was born after his death. Nate was interred at Arlington National Cemetery in Section 60, stone 7978, and was post-humously awarded the Bronze Star with Valor and the Purple Heart.

Please consider making a donation in Nate's name to the Coast Guard Tactical Law Enforcement Foundation. In addition to maintaining an Emergency Assistance Fund for Coast Guard families, they have started a scholarship initiative in Nate's name. Please visit www.CGTLE.org/Scholars to learn more.

BRUCK

4 rounds for time:
RUN (400M)
24 BACK SQUATS (185lbs)
24 JERKS (135lbs)

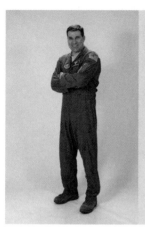

MAJOR
DAVID BRODEUR
April 27, 2011

Photo Credit: FirstGiving.org

David was brought up Auburn, Massachusetts, and set his sights on becoming a pilot early in life. He graduated with honors in 1994 and spent a year at Valley Forge Military Academy before attending the Air Force Academy in Colorado. After earning his political science degree in 1999, David commissioned in the Air Force and qualified as an F-16 fighter pilot. He would become an accomplished aviator, logging over 1,600 flight hours in combat aircraft and flying numerous missions overseas in support of Operation Iraqi Freedom.

While stationed at Eielson Air Force Base in Alaska, he served with the 18th Aggressor Squadron as a flight commander, F-16 instructor, and weapons air defense officer. His next assignment was as the executive officer of the Eleventh Air Force at Joint Base Elmendorf-Richardson in Alaska. David deployed from the unit to Afghanistan as an advisor under NATO Air Training Command. On April 27, 2011, Major David Brodeur, 34, was shot and killed by an Afghan military pilot; seven other service members lost their lives during the attack. David is survived by his widow, Susan; their children, Elizabeth and David Jr.; his parents, Lawrence and Joyce; and his siblings, Todd and Amanda.

The mission of The Major David Brodeur Memorial Foundation is to honor David's life by providing grants to Auburn High School students for academics, athletics, and extra-curricular activities. The foundation hosts the Klepto 5k race annually to help raise funds; to sign up or to make a donation, please visit www.BrodeurFoundation.com.

KLEPTO

4 rounds for time:
27 BOX JUMPS (24")
20 BURPEES
11 SQUAT CLEANS (145lbs)

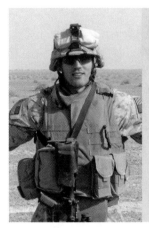

FIRST LIEUTENANT TRAVIS MANION
April 29, 2007

Photo Credit: Crossfitoxnard.com

The Manion family settled in Doylestown, Pennsylvania when Travis was 10. He graduated from LaSalle College High School, and was granted an appointment to the United States Naval Academy in 1999. Travis chose to pursue a career in the Marine Corps, and was assigned to 1st Reconnaissance Battalion, 1st Marine Division at Camp Pendleton, California.

During an eight-month deployment to Iraq, Travis acted with extraordinary courage and was awarded the Bronze Star with Valor. He deployed to Iraq again in late 2006, and was on patrol when his unit was ambushed by insurgents. First Lieutenant Travis Manion, 26, was killed in action on April 29, 2007 by a sniper while engaging the enemy and drawing fire from his wounded teammates. His courage in battle was recognized with the award of a Silver Star and the Purple Heart. Travis is survived by his father, Tom; and his sister, Ryan; his mother, Janet, passed away in 2012. Colonel (Ret.) Tom Manion is the co-author of *Brothers Forever*, which tells the story of Travis and his USNA roommate Brendan Looney, a Navy SEAL who perished in a helicopter crash while deployed overseas. The two are buried next to each other at Arlington National Cemetery, Section 60, stones 9179 and 9180. To read Brendan's story, go to page 212.

The Travis Manion Foundation is dedicated to "honoring the fallen by challenging the living". Their organization assists veterans and families affected by the loss of a military member through support and empowerment programs. Visit their website at www.TravisManion.org.

MANION

7 rounds for time:

RUN (400M)

29 BACK SQUATS (135lbs)

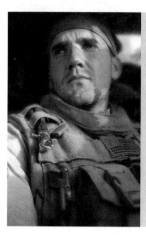

CAPTAIN BRANDON BARRETT
May 5, 2010

Photo Credit: Crossfit-springfield.com

Brandon's family moved to Marion, Indiana when he was nine. He attended Marion High School, and played football and baseball prior to graduating in 2001. From a young age, Brandon voiced aspirations to join the military; he was granted an appointment to the United States Naval Academy, where he chose to pursue a commission in the Marine Corps as an infantry officer. After completing his initial training, Brandon was assigned to 1st Battalion, 6th Marine Regiment, 2nd Marine Division at Camp Lejeune in North Carolina. He deployed to Afghanistan in 2008 to support Operation Enduring Freedom, and was immensely proud of the fact that all of his Marines returned home safely.

Brandon returned to Afghanistan in December 2009 and was sent to the Helmand province. On May 5, 2010, he was working between two armored vehicles, shoveling sand into bags to fortify his unit's position, when an enemy sniper fired two rounds. First Lieutenant Brandon Barrett, 27, was hit in the chest by the first bullet and died of the wound. He leaves behind his parents, Cindy and Brett; his brother, Brock; and his sisters, Ashley and Taylor. Brandon was posthumously promoted to the rank of Captain and, in accordance with his wishes, was laid to rest in Marion.

Founded in 1962, the Marine Corps Scholarship Foundation is dedicated to "honoring Marines by educating their children." To learn more about the scholarship awarded in Brandon's name, please visit www.MCSF.org/Captain-Brandon-Barrett-USMC.

BULL

2 rounds for time:

200 DOUBLE-UNDERS

50 OVERHEAD SQUATS (135lbs)

50 PULL-UPS

RUN (1 MILE)

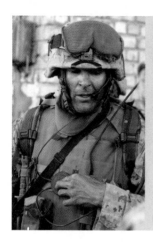

MAJOR DOUGLAS ZEMBIEC
May 11, 2007

Photo Credit: Archive.defense.gov

Doug was raised in Albuquerque, and attended the Naval Academy to commission with the Marine Corps in 1995. He completed deployments to Kosovo and Iraq and, in 2004, was serving as the commander of Company E, 2nd Battalion, 1st Marine Regiment when he became known as "the Lion of Fallujah". A Marine told Doug's father, "I was with your son [in Iraq]…If we had to go back in there, I would follow him with a spoon."

Doug was selected for a billet with the Ground Branch of the CIA's Special Activities Division. On May 11, 2007, he was leading a team on a mission in Baghdad when he realized they were about to be ambushed. Major Douglas Zembiec, 34, called out in warning but was shot in the head and killed moments later. He is survived by his widow, Pamela; their daughter, Fallyn; his parents, Donald and Jo Ann; and his brother, John. Doug was interred at Arlington National Cemetery in Section 60, stone 8621, and was posthumously awarded the Silver Star. Though it remains listed in anonymity, the only star the CIA inscribed in the Memorial Wall for 2007 was in honor of Doug. Please consider reading *Selfless Beyond Service* by Pamela Zembiec to learn more about Doug and the standards he set as a leader.

Marine Corps Scholarship Foundation has endowed the Major Doug Zembiec USMC and Major Ray Mendoza USMC Memorial Scholarship to honor two friends who both gave their lives in Iraq. To make a donation, please go to www.MCSF.org.

ZEMBIEC

5 rounds for time:
11 BACK SQUATS (185lbs)
7 BURPEE PULL-UPS*
RUN (400M)

Workout Notes
*Strict—no kipping
Bar 12" above max standing reach

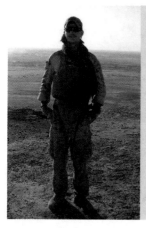

SERGEANT WADE WILSON
May 11, 2012

Photo Credit: Crossfit

Wade "Willy" Wilson was a native of a small Texas town called Leona. At the age of 17, he enlisted in the Marine Corps and left for boot camp just after his graduation in 2007. Willy trained as an infantryman and served two tours of duty overseas before reporting to Camp Pendleton, California. He was assigned to 2nd Battalion, 5th Marine Regiment, 1st Marine Division and deployed with the unit to Afghanistan as the platoon sergeant of 3rd Platoon, Weapons Company.

On May 11, 2012, Willy was providing security for an armored vehicle when it was disabled by an improvised explosive device; an insurgent began firing an AK-47 and hit one of the Marines inside. Willy immediately drew his service pistol and moved toward the enemy, placing himself directly between the other Marines and the gunman. Sergeant Wade Wilson, 22, returned fire until he fell, mortally wounded. He is survived by his mother and stepfather, Cindy Lee and Ward Easterling; his father and stepmother, Mitchell Boyd and Tammy Wilson; his brothers, Chad, Alex, and Curtis; his sister, Layne; and his stepsisters, Teri, Amy, and Lisa. Willy's actions saved the lives of his fellow Marines; for his courage under fire, he was posthumously decorated with the Silver Star and the Purple Heart.

At his funeral, Willy's family requested donations in his name be made to a charity he believed in and regularly donated to, St. Jude Children's Research Hospital. Please visit them at www.StJude.org.

WILLY

3 rounds for time:

RUN (800M)

5 FRONT SQUATS (225lbs)

RUN (200M)

11 CHEST-TO-BAR PULL-UPS

RUN (400M)

12 KB SWINGS (2 pood)

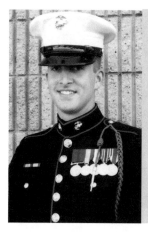

SERGEANT JOSHUA DESFORGES
May 12, 2010

Photo Credit: Thefallen.militarytimes.com

Josh was raised in Ludlow, Massachusetts, and began participating in the Westover Young Marines at the age of 13. He enlisted shortly after graduating high school in 2004 and went through boot camp at Parris Island, South Carolina. After finishing the School of Infantry, Josh was assigned to 1st Battalion, 6th Marine Regiment, 2nd Marine Division at Camp Lejeune in North Carolina. He deployed to Afghanistan for the first time in 2008, and returned for a second tour in December of the next year.

Now a squad leader, Josh worked diligently to build relationships with the locals; he even asked his mother to gather school supplies for the Afghan children in Marjah. On 12, 2010, Sergeant Joshua Desforges, 23, was shot and killed during combat operations. He is survived by his parents, David and Arlene; and his sister, Janelle. Josh's body was escorted home by Sergeant Major (Ret.) Edward Mitrook, his leader from the Westover Young Marines. Josh was also posthumously decorated with the Purple Heart.

In Ludlow, Josh was the first resident service member to die in combat since the Vietnam War; a memorial dedicated to him stands in front of Ludlow High School, and bears the words "Honor. Courage. Commitment." The school also hosts an annual fitness challenge to raise funds for scholarships awarded in Josh's name. To sign up for the event or to make a donation, please go to www.LudlowPS.org and select the tab marked "Sgt. Joshua D. Desforges, USMC."

DESFORGES

5 rounds for time:

12 DEADLIFTS (225lbs)

20 PULL-UPS

12 CLEAN AND JERKS (135lbs)

20 KNEES-TO-ELBOWS

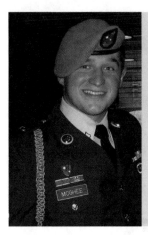

CORPORAL RYAN MCGHEE
May 13, 2009

Photo Credit: Arlingtoncemetery.net

Ryan grew up in Vermont and moved to Fredericksburg, Virginia during his sophomore year of high school. He became a standout football player at Massaponax High School, but turned down a college athletic scholarship to enlist in the Army in 2006. Ryan had idolized Arizona Cardinals player Pat Tillman, and much as Tillman had, Ryan was determined to become a Ranger, completing the Ranger Indoctrination Program in 2007.

While assigned to 3rd Battalion, 75th Ranger Regiment at Fort Benning, Ryan served three tours of duty in Afghanistan as a rifleman and grenadier. He then deployed to Iraq as a weapons squad team leader, and his unit was tasked with eliminating a suicide-bombing cell and weapons provider. On May 13, 2009, Corporal Ryan McGhee, 21, was engaging the enemy and helping to move civilians out of harm's way when a ricocheting bullet struck under his armor; he continued to return fire until he succumbed to the wound. Ryan is survived by his fiancée, Ashleigh Mitchell; his mother, Sherrie Battle-McGhee; his father and stepmother, Steven and Kristie McGhee; and his brother, Zachary. He was interred at Arlington National Cemetery in Section 60, stone 8870, and posthumously awarded the Bronze Star with Valor and the Purple Heart.

Ryan's high school holds an annual memorial game to honor him and other veterans in their community, with donations benefiting Warrior 360. The organization's mission is to rapidly respond in times of crisis for service members and their families. To learn more, please visit www.Warrior360.org.

MCGHEE

In 30 minutes, as many rounds as possible:

5 DEADLIFTS (275lbs)

13 PUSH-UPS

9 BOX JUMPS (24")

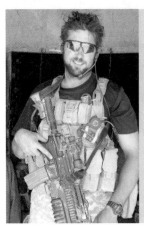

STAFF SERGEANT JOSH WHITAKER

May 15, 2007

Photo Credit: Crossfit

Josh was raised in Long Beach, California and grew up close to his two younger cousins, Rachel and Laura. After graduating high school in 2003, he enlisted in the Army to pursue a career in Special Forces. Josh earned his Green Beret nearly three years later and reported to 1st Battalion, 7th Special Forces Group (Airborne) at Fort Bragg, North Carolina. As a Special Forces engineer sergeant, Josh had found his calling: a fellow staff sergeant later described him as "rock-hard Soldier" who "really loved to blow things up".

Josh's twenty-third birthday was March 10, 2007—the same day he deployed to Afghanistan. On May 15, his team was returning from a mission when their convoy was attacked in an ambush. Staff Sergeant Joshua Whitaker was manning the .50 caliber turret gun and laying down cover for the other vehicles when he was fatally struck by enemy fire. He is survived by his mother, Cathy; his uncle and aunt, Robb and Debbie; his cousins, Rachel and Laura; his girlfriend, Star Boyd; and his father, Frank Dougherty. Josh was posthumously given a number of awards, amongst them the Bronze Star with Valor, the Purple Heart, and the Combat Infantryman Badge.

Laura, Josh's youngest cousin, was diagnosed with diabetes at nine years old. Josh had sat with her, testing his own blood sugar to show her it was no big deal. His family suggested donations in his name be made to the Juvenile Diabetes Research Foundation; to learn more about their work, please visit www.JDRF.org.

JOSHIE

3 rounds for time:

21 DUMBBELL SNATCHES (40lbs) RIGHT ARM

21 L PULL-UPS

21 DUMBBELL SNATCHES (40lbs) LEFT ARM

21 L PULL-UPS

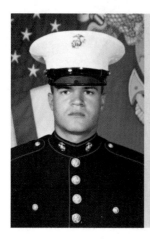

LANCE CORPORAL PHILIP CLARK
May 18, 2010

Photo Credit: Thefallen.militarytimes.com

Born in Mississippi, Philip grew up in Florida and attended Buchholz High School in Gainesville. He set his sights on joining the Marine Corps, and spent his senior year preparing himself for boot camp. Shortly after graduating in 2008, Philip entered basic training at Parris Island in South Carolina. He was subsequently stationed with 1st Battalion, 6th Marine Regiment, 2nd Marine Division at Camp Lejeune, North Carolina and deployed with the unit in December of 2009.

Philip was a jokester who knew how to make people laugh. He was also a patriot with an innate drive to lead, and was completely dedicated to his team. Though he had qualified for a position as a sniper, Philip declined in order to stay with his platoon, and often took point position at the front of the squad during patrols. On May 18, Lance Corporal Philip Clark was struck by the blast of an improvised explosive device and died of his wounds soon after. He is survived by his widow, Ashton; his parents, Mike and Tammy Clark; his mother, Rosmari Kruger; and his brothers, Tyler, Kyle, and Ryan Nordyke. Philip was laid to rest with full military honors and his family was presented with his Purple Heart.

Philip's family requested donations in his name be made to the Community Foundation of North Central Florida. The CFNCF maintains the Philip Paul Clark Scholarship Fund and awards tuition to JAFROTC students at Buchholz High School. To make a donation, please visit www.CFNCF.org.

PHEEZY

3 rounds for time:
5 FRONT SQUATS (165lbs)
18 PULL-UPS
5 DEADLIFTS (225lbs)
18 TOES-TO-BAR
5 PUSH JERKS (165lbs)
18 HAND-RELEASE PUSH-UPS

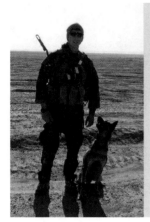

CORPORAL KEATON COFFEY
May 24, 2012

Photo Credit: Crossfit

Keaton lived in the town of Boring his entire life and attended Damascus Christian School from kindergarten through high school. After graduating in 2007, he began taking classes at George Fox University but chose to enlist in the Marine Corps after two semesters. Keaton completed training for military police officers before reporting to Camp Pendleton, California and, in 2010, volunteered for a seven-month tour of duty in Afghanistan. Hewas then accepted into K9 School to become a Military Working Dog Handler, and deployed back to Afghanistan with Denny, a German shepherd, in December 2011.

Keaton was engaged to be married, his wedding date just weeks after he was due home. When his contract with the Marines was fulfilled, Keaton wanted to continue his education and become a firefighter, like his father. On May 24, 2012, Corporal Keaton Coffey, 22, was mortally wounded by enemy sniper fire while conducting combat operations in the Helmand province of Afghanistan. He is survived by his fiancée, Brittany Dygert; his parents, Grant and Inger; and his canine partner, Denny.

The Keaton Coffey Memorial Scholarship Fund was established to provide financial assistance to students enrolled at Damascus Christian School. To make a donation, please visit www.DCEF4You.org. The Hero Half, an annual half-marathon, was also founded to honor Keaton's memory; proceeds from the race benefit his scholarship fund and a local chapter of the Vietnam Veterans of America. Online race registration is available at www.HeroHalf.org.

COFFEY

For time:

RUN (800M)

50 BACK SQUATS (135lbs)

50 BENCH PRESSES (135lbs)

RUN (800M)

35 BACK SQUATS (135lbs)

35 BENCH PRESSES (135lbs)

RUN (800M)

20 BACK SQUATS (135lbs)

20 BENCH PRESSES (135lbs)

RUN (800M)

1 MUSCLE-UP

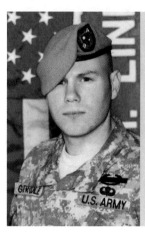

SPECIALIST CHRISTOPHER GATHERCOLE
May 26, 2008

Photo Credit: Crossfit

Chris had a rougher start in life than many. Born in Santa Rosa, California, he spent the majority of his childhood in the foster care system of Sonoma County. As he approached graduation at Rincon High School in Carpinteria, Chris committed to joining the military and enlisted in the Army in October 2005. He completed Basic Combat Training and Infantry School at Fort Benning, Georgia followed by the Basic Airborne Course and the Ranger Indoctrination Program. In keeping with his tenacious nature, Chris earned his Ranger tab in May 2006 and was subsequently stationed as a lightweight machine gunner with 2nd Battalion, 75th Ranger Regiment at Fort Lewis, Washington.

On May 26, 2008, Specialist Christopher Gathercole, 21, was killed by enemy small arms fire during combat operations in Ghazni, Afghanistan. He is survived by his siblings, Edward Gathercole, Jennifer Daly, and Sarah Ferrell; his mother, Catherine Haines; and his father, Edward Gathercole. Chris was buried with full military honors and was posthumously awarded the Bronze Star with Valor, the Purple Heart, the Meritorious Service Medal, and the Army Good Conduct Medal.

If you would like to make a contribution in memory of Chris, please consider the Court Appointed Special Advocates of Sonoma County, whose volunteers made such an impact on his life. The program supports children in foster care by assigning them an advocate, who is dedicated to their case and can provide additional representation on their behalf in court. To learn more or make a contribution, visit www.SonomaCASA.org.

GATOR

8 rounds for time:
5 FRONT SQUATS (185lbs)
26 RING PUSH-UPS

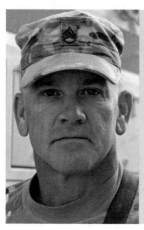

STAFF SERGEANT ALEXANDER POVILAITIS
May 31, 2012

Photo Credit: Crossfit

Alexander first enlisted in the Army when he was 18, and served for three years as a radio operator. After completing his commitment, Alexander returned to his home state of Georgia to work in construction; he would later work on landmark projects, including Centennial Olympic Park, the Mall of Georgia, and Turner Field. In 2008, Alexander returned to serve in the Army and qualified as a combat engineer. He then reported to White Sands Missile Range in New Mexico and served a tour of duty in support of Operation Iraqi Freedom. Alexander next received orders in 2011 to Joint Base Lewis-McChord, Washington with 570th Sapper Company, 14th Engineer Battalion, 555th Engineer Brigade. That year, he deployed to Afghanistan as a squad leader in 2nd Platoon.

Staff Sergeant Alexander Povilaitis, 47, was killed on May 31, 2012 in Kandahar province when an improvised explosive device detonated during a route clearance mission. He is survived by his widow, Kimberley; his sons, David and Blaine; his stepchildren, Zach, Shane, Kyle, and Kaitlyn; and his father, Alexander Povilaitis, Sr. Alexander was posthumously decorated with the Bronze Star and the Purple Heart in recognition of his sacrifice.

Please consider making a contribution in Alexander's name to the Iraq and Afghanistana Veterans of America, an organization dedicated to supporting and empowering veterans and their families. Read more about their current intiatives and programs at iava.org.

ALEXANDER

5 rounds for time:

31 BACK SQUATS (135lbs)
12 POWER CLEANS (185lbs)

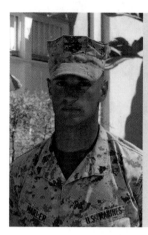

CORPORAL DONALD MARLER
June 6, 2010

Photo Credit: Crossfit

Don was from Oakville, a town just south of St. Louis in Missouri. He decided early on that he would enlist in the Marine Corps, and famously missed his own high school commencement ceremony to attend boot camp at the first opportunity. After an assignment to the Presidential Security Detail at Camp David, Don was eager to serve overseas and requested orders to 3rd Battalion, 1st Marine Regiment, 1st Marine Division; the unit was already scheduled to deploy to the Helmand province of Afghanistan in April 2010.

In spite of his assignment to Headquarters and Service Company, Don volunteered for every patrol and convoy he could. On June 6, Corporal Donald Marler, 22, was manning the turret gunner position of an armored vehicle when it rolled into a canal; all three Marines inside were unable to escape and drowned. Don is survived by his parents, Susan and David Sr.; his sister Jennifer; his brothers, David Jr. and Jacob; and his girlfriend, Joelle Keams.

When Don's body arrived in St. Louis, the city turned out in force to pay their respects. I-55 South was shut down for the procession; the overpasses were lined by hundreds of people, and a giant American flag hung over the highway. In lieu of flowers at his funeral, Don's family requested donations in his name be made to the Fisher House. Read more about how they support military service members and their families at www.FisherHouse.org.

THE DON

For time:

66 DEADLIFTS (110lbs)

66 BOX JUMPS (24")

66 KB SWINGS (1.5 pood)

66 KNEES-TO-ELBOWS

66 SIT-UPS

66 PULL-UPS

66 THRUSTERS (55lbs)

66 WALL BALL SHOTS (20lbs)

66 BURPEES

66 DOUBLE-UNDERS

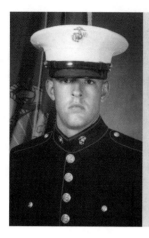

SERGEANT JOHN RANKEL
June 7, 2010

Photo Credit: Goldstarfamilyregistry.com

John spent the last five years of his life proudly serving in the Marine Corps. After his graduation in 2005 from Speedway High School in Indianapolis, John chose to enlist and went on to complete two tours of duty in Iraq. He later received orders to 3rd Battalion, 1st Marine Regiment, 1st Marine Division at Camp Pendleton, and deployed to Afghanistan as a squad leader in 2010.

During a patrol in on June 7, a number of John's Marines began taking fire with only haystacks to shield them. He didn't hesitate to run through machine gun fire and rocket-propelled grenades to get to their position, and proceeded to exchange fire with the enemy while the other men fell back. Having assured the safety of his fellow Marines, Sergeant John Rankel, 23, was returning to cover when he was shot in the chest; he was pulled from harm's way to await a CASEVAC helicopter, but did not survive the wound. John leaves behind his mother and stepfather, Trisha and Don Stockhoff; his father and stepmother, Kevin and Kim Rankel; his brothers, Tyler Rankel and Nathan Stockoff; and his girlfriend, Lindsay Raikes. For his bravery in the face of the enemy, John was posthumously awarded the Bronze Star with Valor and the Purple Heart.

The Marine Corps Scholarship Foundation maintains memorial scholarships in the names of fallen Marines, including John. Their focus is providing tuition to the children of Marines and Navy Corpsmen who were killed or wounded in combat; to make a donation in John's name, please visit www.MCSF.org.

RANKEL

In 20 minutes, as many rounds as possible:

6 DEADLIFTS (225lbs)

7 BURPEE PULL-UPS

10 KB SWINGS (2 pood)

RUN (200M)

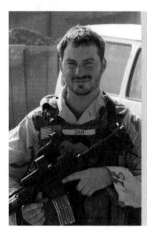

SERGEANT FIRST CLASS DANIEL CRABTREE

June 8, 2006

Photo Credit: Crossfitnewengland.com

Daniel was raised in Hartville, Ohio and joined the Army Reserve in 1992 through an early enlistment program. After graduating from Lake High School the following year, he entered service with the Army National Guard. Daniel earned his associate's degree in criminal justice from the University of Akron and spent a year working for his hometown police force. He then transferred to the nearby town of Cuyahoga Falls and served as a member of their SWAT unit.

In 2003, Daniel was sent to the Special Forces Qualification Course and earned his Green Beret the following year. He completed tours of duty to Iraq and Nicaragua during his military service, and deployed for a second time to Iraq with Ohio National Guard Company B, 2nd Battalion, 19th Special Forces Group (Airborne). As the lead trainer for the Iraqi Police Force in Al Kut, Daniel's prior experience helped him form one of the most effective local police units in Iraq. On June 8, 2006, Sergeant First Class Daniel Crabtree, 31, was critically wounded by the detonation of a roadside bomb near his vehicle and died his wounds en route to a combat support hospital. Daniel is survived by his widow, Kathy; their daughter, Mallory; his mother, Judy Ann; and his father, Donald. He was posthumously awarded the Bronze Star and the Purple Heart, amongst other decorations.

The community of Cuyahoga Falls holds an annual 5k race to honor Daniel and benefit the Special Operations Warrior Foundation; please visit www.Crabtree MemorialRun.org for more information.

DANIEL

For time:

50 PULL-UPS

RUN (400M)

21 THRUSTERS (95lbs)

RUN (800M)

21 THRUSTERS (95lbs)

RUN (400M)

50 PULL-UPS

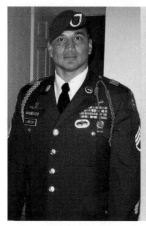

STAFF SERGEANT EDWARDO LOREDO
June 24, 2010

Photo Credit: Crosstownathletics.com

Eddie grew up in Houston and graduated from Sam Houston High School. Without telling anyone, he enlisted in the Army in 1999 and began training for the airborne infantry. Eddie was initially stationed in Italy with 1st Battalion, 508th Parachute Infantry Regiment, 173rd Brigade Combat Team (Airborne) and deployed to Iraq in 2003. After a year spent working with the 663rd Movement Control Team, he rejoined 1st Battalion and completed a tour of duty in Afghanistan. Eddie was then assigned to Company F, 51st Infantry (Long Range Surveillance) at Fort Bragg, North Carolina and returned to Iraq for 14-months. In October 2009, he received his final orders to 2nd Battalion, 508th Parachute Regiment, 4th Brigade Combat Team, 82nd Airborne Division and began preparing for another deployment to Afghanistan.

On June 24, 2010, Staff Sergeant Edward Loredo, 34, was patrolling with his unit when he was fatally injured by the detonation of an improvised explosive device. Eddie is survived by his widow, Master Sergeant Jennifer Loredo; his son, Eduardo; his daughter, Laura; his stepdaughter, Alexis; and his brothers, Sylvester, Alfredo, and Angel. He was interred at Arlington National Cemetery in Section 60, stone 9169, and was posthumously decorated with the Bronze Star and the Purple Heart.

To make a donation in Eddie's memory, please consider the Fisher House Foundation. Since 1991, they have provided assistance to injured Soldiers and their families to facilitate their recovery. Please visit them at www.FisherHouse.org.

<u>LOREDO</u>

6 rounds for time:
24 SQUATS
24 PUSH-UPS
24 WALKING LUNGE STEPS
RUN (400M)

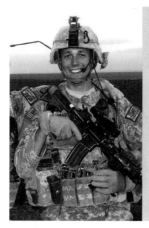

FIRST LIEUTENANT BRIAN BRADSHAW

June 25, 2009

Photo Credit: Crossfit

Brian believed that service is the foundation of life, and lived accordingly. Growing up in Steilacoom, Washington, he was an accomplished outdoorsman who skied and climbed mountains, and served as a member of the Pierce County Search and Rescue. After graduating from Bellarimine High School, Brian began pursuing his political science degree at Pacific Lutheran University and became a cadet in the Army ROTC program. He commissioned as an infantry officer in 2007 and was sent to Fort Benning, where he completed the Basic Airborne Course and earned his Ranger tab. He was then assigned as a platoon leader to 1st Battalion, 501st Parachute Infantry Regiment, 4th Airborne Brigade Combat Team, 25th Infantry Division at Fort Richardson, Alaska.

On June 25, 2009, First Lieutenant Brian Bradshaw, 24, was killed by the blast of an improvised explosive device while on patrol in Afghanistan. He is survived by his parents, Paul and Mary; and his brother, Robert. During his military service, Brian had truly earned the respect of his men. A letter was written to Brian's family by two members of the crew that escorted his body to Bagram Air Base; in it, they detailed the reverence with which Brian was treated, how "…the war stopped to honor Lt. Brian Bradshaw."

Brian was committed to education: he said it changes how we treat people, how we see the world. Pacific Lutheran University maintains an endowed scholarship in his name; to make a contribution, please visit the university's giving page at www.PLU.edu/Advancement.

BRADSHAW

10 rounds for time:

3 HANDSTAND PUSH-UPS

6 DEADLIFTS (225lbs)

12 PULL-UPS

24 DOUBLE-UNDERS

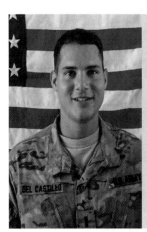

FIRST LIEUTENANT DIMITRI DEL CASTILLO
June 25, 2011

Photo Credit: Letronocrossfit.com

Del graduated from James E. Taylor High School in Katy, Texas. He was granted an appointment to the United States Military Academy at West Point and spent his junior year abroad studying in Spain. In 2009, Del commissioned as an infantry officer and went to Fort Benning, Georgia to earn his Ranger tab and Airborne wings. He then received orders to 2nd Battalion, 35th Infantry Regiment, 3rd Brigade Combat Team, 25th Infantry Division at Schofield Barracks, Hawaii.

Del deployed in April 2011 to the Kunar province of Afghanistan as the platoon leader of 1st Platoon, Company B. On June 25, he was leading his soldiers on a mission to locate and destroy insurgents when they came under attack. First Lieutenant Dimitri del Castillo, 24, was fatally wounded by enemy small arms fire while radioing back for support; the attack took the life of one other Soldier. Del is survived by his widow, Katie; his parents, Carlos and Catherine; and his siblings, Carlos, Andres, and Anna. He was laid to rest at West Point alongside his friend and classmate First Lieutenant Daren Hidalgo, whose story can be found on page 28. For his bravery, Del was posthumously awarded the Bronze Star and the Purple Heart.

The U.S. Army Ranger Association maintains the First Lieutenant Dimitri del Castillo Scholarship, which is offered annually to the child or spouse of a fallen Ranger. To make a donation, please visit www.Ranger.org and select the tab labeled "USARA Scholarship Program".

DEL

For time:

25 BURPEES

RUN (400M)*

25 WEIGHTED PULL-UPS**

RUN (400M)*

25 HANDSTAND PUSH-UPS

RUN (400M)*

25 CHEST-TO-BAR PULL-UPS

RUN (400M)*

25 BURPEES

Workout Notes
*With a 20lbs medicine ball
**With a 20lbs dumbbell

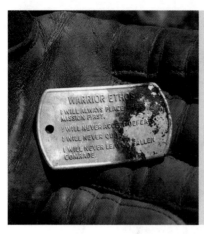

OPERATION RED WINGS
June 28, 2005

Photo Credit: Abcnews.com

Late on the night of June 27, 2005, four SEALs were inserted into the Hindu Kush Mountains of Afghanistan. They moved on foot through the forests of the Kunar province; their assignment was to locate Ahmad Shah, a terrorist leader aligned with the Taliban. The mission was compromised when the team was spotted by locals, who reported their location to anti-coalition forces. Shortly after, the SEALs were engaged by a militant force with mortars, rocket-propelled grenades, and small-arms fire. Communications in the mountains were unreliable at best. In order to transmit his team's position back to the Quick Reaction Force at Bagram Air Base, Lieutenant Michael Murphy knowingly exposed himself to enemy fire and was shot multiple times.

After receiving the call for troops in contact, eight SEALs and eight Night Stalkers quickly boarded a MH-47 Chinook helicopter to retrieve the entrenched team. The Chinook soon outran its escort of heavily-armored Army attack helicopters; in the light of day, the transport helicopter was vulnerable and exposed. When the rescue team arrived on site, the Chinook hovered as the SEALs prepared to fast-rope down to the mountainous terrain. Suddenly, a rocket-propelled grenade was launched and struck the helicopter, killing all 16 men on board.

On the ground, three of the four SEALs were dead. It was not until July 4 that the recovery team was able to locate and bring home the bodies of the fallen Night Stalkers and SEALs.

The remaining man, Petty Officer First Class Marcus Luttrell, had been shot and was severely injured. He dragged himself further down the mountain and evaded Taliban forces before he was found by a shepherd named Gulab. The man took Marcus to his village, where he was kept safely for several days in spite of threats from the Taliban. Another villager couriered a note from Marcus to a Marine outpost and a rescue mission was launched. Marcus was recovered by American Forces on July 3. He was awarded the Navy Cross and the Purple Heart for his actions during Operation Red Wings and returned to serve with the SEAL Team FIVE. In 2007, he medically retired after completing a tour of duty in Iraq.

With the help of author Patrick Robinson, Marcus published his account of Operation Red Wing, titled *Lone Survivor*; the book was made into a major motion picture and released in 2013. After leaving active duty, Marcus started the Lone Survivor Foundation. The organization is dedicated to helping wounded service members and their families through programs aimed at recovery. To make a contribution, please visit www.LoneSurvivorFoundation.org.

The 160th Special Operations Aviation Regiment (Airborne) was formed in 1981 after a failed rescue attempt during the Iranian hostage Crisis. The Night Stalkers specialize in nighttime missions, and have participated in every Army combat action since their founding. The Soldiers of the 160th live fiercely by their motto, "Night Stalkers Don't Quit." At Hunter Army Airfield in Georgia, the regiment renamed their Chinook hangar in honor of the eight Night Stalkers they lost during Operation Red Wings: it now bears the name Turbine 33, after the downed crew's call sign. Hangar Turbine 33 was entered into the National Archives as an Army memorial, and the call sign has been retired from use.

In making donations in honor of Operation Red Wings, please also consider the Night Stalker Association. For over 25 years, they have provided assistance to Night Stalkers and their families while preserving the memory of their fallen members. Please visit them at www.NSA160.com.

OPERATION RED WINGS

4 rounds for time:

3 BARBELL COMPLEXES (110/75LBS)

RUN (800M)

8 BARBELL BURPEES (110/75LBS)

RUN (800M)

8 THRUSTERS (110/75LBS)

RUN (800M)

Courtesy of CrossFit Fire
McHenry, Illinois

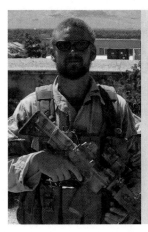

PETTY OFFICER SECOND CLASS MATTHEW AXELSON

Photo Credit: Wikipedia.org

Matt graduated from Monte Vista High School in Cupertino, California in 1994. He earned his degree in political science from California State University in Chico before enlisting in the Navy in December 2000. After initial training as a sonar technician, Matt entered the pipeline to become a SEAL and, in 2002, reported to his first duty station at SEAL Delivery Vehicle Team ONE in Pearl Harbor, Hawaii.

On June 28, 2005, Matt was a member of the four-man reconnaissance team hunting a Taliban leader in the mountains of Afghanistan. During the battle that ensued between the SEALs and the insurgent force, Matt fought long beyond what most would consider humanly possible. He suffered shots to the head and chest, and was hit by the blast of a rocket-propelled grenade. Petty Officer Second Class Matthew Axelson, 29, continued to fire his weapon at the enemy until he succumbed to his wounds. His last words, spoken to Petty Officer Luttrell, were, "…tell Cindy I love her." He leaves behind his widow, Cindy; his parents, Cordell and Donna; and his brother, Jeffrey. For the extreme courage he displayed in the mountains of Afghanistan, Matt was posthumously awarded the Navy Cross.

Jeffrey Axelson is the author of Matt's biography, *Axe: A Brother's Search for an American Warrior, Navy SEAL Matthew Axelson*. He and Cindy also maintain the Matthew Axelson Foundation, which provides aid to active duty service members and veteran families. To learn more about their initiatives, please visit www.MatthewAxelsonFoundation.org.

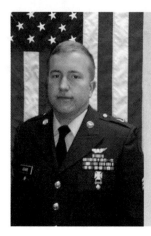

STAFF SERGEANT SHAMUS GOARE

Photo Credit: Iraqwarheroes

Shamus grew up in Danville, Ohio. In 1994, he infamously tricked his mother into signing the paperwork that would allow him to enlist at 17 years old. Shamus' parents thought he might get to see the world before starting college, but that wasn't the case: he went on to serve in the Army for 11 years. He began his career as a Huey helicopter repairer, and in 1996 was assigned to Sinai, Egypt as a Huey crew chief. After a year overseas, Shamus spent another tour working as a crew chief at Fort Belvoir in Virginia. He then completed the Heavy Helicopter Repairer Course and was stationed at Camp Humphreys in Korea to repair Chinook Helicopters. In 2000, Shamus joined 3rd Battalion, 160th Special Operations Aviation Regiment (Airborne), based at Hunter Army Airfield in Georgia.

On June 28, 2005, Staff Sergeant Shamus Goare, 29, gave his life while serving as a flight engineer on board the downed Chinook helicopter. He is survived by his parents, Judith and Charles; and his brother, Kortney. Shamus was decorated posthumously with a number of awards, including the Bronze Star, the Purple Heart, and Air Medal with Valor.

Shamus' funeral procession through the streets of Danville was led by six vintage hot rods—one of Shamus' favorite things. In lieu of flowers, Shamus' family requested donations be made in his name to the Night Stalkers Association.

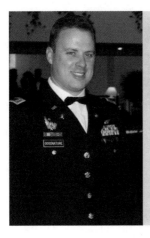

CHIEF WARRANT OFFICER 3 COREY GOODNATURE

Photo Credit: Coreygoodnature.com

Corey was raised in Clarks Grove, Minnesota. He began attending the University of Minnesota as a ROTC cadet in 1988, but lost his entry options to both Air Force and Marine Corps aviation when the school's military programs began suffering from cutbacks. Determined to fly, Corey chose instead to enlist in the Army and left the university with his associate's degree in aerospace engineering.

Before he was accepted to flight school, Corey spent four years working as parachute rigger at the John F. Kennedy Special Warfare Center and School at Fort Bragg. He became an aviator in 1995, deploying three times to Afghanistan and once to Iraq. He was selected for Special Operations in 1998, and stationed at Hunter Army Air Field in Georgia to fly Chinook helicopters with 3rd Battalion, 160th Special Operations Aviation Regiment (Airborne).

On June 28, 2005, Chief Warrant Officer 3 Corey Goodnature, 34, was serving as the flight lead pilot of the Chinook helicopter. He is survived by his widow, Lori; his sons, Shea and Brennan; his parents, Don and Deb; and his sister, Amy. In recognition of his service, Corey was decorated posthumously with a number of awards, including the Bronze Star, the Purple Heart, and the Air Medal with Valor.

The Corey Goodnature Memorial Scholarship Fund provides scholarships to students living near Corey's hometown in Minnesota; the organization also makes contributions to the Night Stalker Association. To learn more, please visit www.CoreyGoodnature.com.

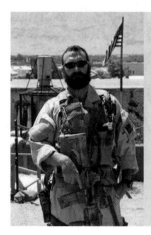

SENIOR CHIEF PETTY OFFICER DANIEL HEALY

Photo Credit: Findagrave.com

Dan was a native of Exeter, New Hampshire and graduated from Exeter High School in 1986. Four years later, he enlisted in the Navy and entered Basic Underwater Demolition/SEAL training in January 1991. Dan was first assigned to SEAL Delivery Vehicle Team ONE based in Pearl Harbor, Hawaii and served with the unit until December 1996. He received a year of language instruction before transferring to SEAL Delivery Vehicle Team TWO in Little Creek, Virginia. After six months six months deployed aboard the USS Ponce (LPD-15), Dan returned to SDVT-1 in March 2000 and remained with the unit for the duration of his service.

On June 28, 2005, Dan insisted on taking a seat in the lead Chinook; he said, "Those are my men and my face is going to be the first one they see." Senior Chief Petty Officer Daniel Healy, 36, lost his life when the Chinook was shot down by a rocket-propelled grenade. He is survived by his widow, Norminda; his children, Chelsea, Jake, Jasmine, and Sasha; his mother, Natalie; his father, Tom; his sisters, Jennifer and Shannon; and his half-siblings, Sean and Carrie. In recognition of his courageous service, Dan was posthumously awarded the Bronze Star with Valor and the Purple Heart.

In 2015, the Dan Healy Inaugural Veterans Matter 5k Run/Walk was held to raise funds for the Lone Survivor Foundation and the Dan Healy Foundation. To read more about the event and their mission, please visit www.TheDanHealyFoundation.org.

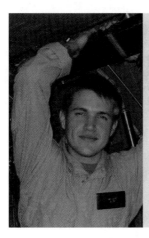

SERGEANT KIP JACOBY

Photo Credit: Gazingattheflag.com

Kip was raised in Pompano Beach, Florida and graduated from Northeast High School in 2002. That October, he enlisted in the Army and began training as a heavy helicopter repairman. Kip received orders in May 2003 to the 160th Special Aviation Operations Regiment Training Company; after completing the Basic Mission Qualification Course, he was stationed with 3rd Battalion, 160th Special Operations Aviation Regiment (Airborne) at Hunter Army Airfield in Georgia. In 2004, Kip was assigned as a flight engineer to Company B and began deploying to the Middle East. During 2004 and 2005, he completed multiple tours of duty in Iraq and Afghanistan in support of Operations Iraqi Freedom and Enduring Freedom.

On June 28, 2005, Sergeant Kip Jacoby, 21, was working as a flight engineer aboard the Chinook when it was shot down by enemy fire. He is survived by his parents, Stephen and Susan Jacoby. For his sacrifice, Kip was posthumously awarded a number of decorations including the Bronze Star, the Purple Heart, and the Air Medal with Valor.

In 2015, the 1st Annual Sgt. Kip A. Jacoby Memorial Kookout was held to raise funds for a music scholarship at Northeast High School in Kip's name. For more information on future events, please visit the "Sgt. Kip A. Jacoby Kookout" Facebook page.

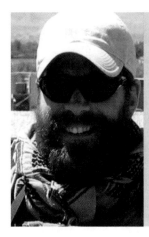

LIEUTENANT COMMANDER ERIK KRISTENSEN

Photo Credit: Pritzkermilitary.org

Erik was not what many people would consider a "typical Navy SEAL." He was a prolific reader and talented writer, spoke French, played the trumpet, and often wore Birkenstocks. In 1995, Erik earned his English degree from the United States Naval Academy and commissioned as a surface warfare officer. He served two years aboard the USS Chandler (DDG-996), then received orders to Special Boat Team TWELVE. Erik returned to Annapolis in 1999 to pursue his graduate degree at St. John's College while teaching English at the Naval Academy.

A year later Erik was granted a lateral transfer to Special Warfare; at 27, he was the oldest graduate of his BUD/S class. Erik spent the next four years working with SEAL Teams EIGHT and TEN and, in 2005, deployed to Afghanistan with SEAL Team TEN as their task unit commander. He was alerted to the plight of his fellow SEALs and organized the rescue mission on June 28. Disregarding his seniority in rank, Lieutenant Commander Erik Kristensen, 33, insisted on leading his team directly and was on board the Chinook when it was shot down. He is survived by his parents, Edward and Suzanne, and was posthumously decorated with the Bronze Star with Valor, the Purple Heart, and several other awards. Erik was laid to rest at the Naval Academy Cemetery in his Birkenstocks.

The Erik Kristensen Eye Street Klassic is a charity golf event held annually to raise funds for a scholarship given in Erik's name. Visit the event site at www.Kristensen Klassic.com.

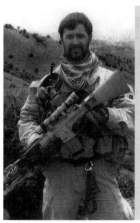

PETTY OFFICER FIRST CLASS JEFFREY LUCAS

Photo Credit: Veterantributes.com

In the fourth grade, Jeff wrote a paper about Special Forces and decided he was going to be a Navy SEAL. He grew up in the town of Corbett, Oregon and enlisted in the Navy after graduating high school in 1989. Originally trained as an electronics technician, Jeff worked at duty stations in Hawaii and California before entering Basic Underwater Demolition/SEAL training in June 1993. He went on to serve with SEAL Team ONE, the Naval Special Warfare Development Group, SEAL Team EIGHT, and Naval Special Warfare Unit TWO. During his career, Jeff deployed overseas numerous times and served in Sri Lanka, Kosovo, and the Philippines. He received his final set of orders to SEAL Team TEN and deploy with the unit to Afghanistan in 2005.

On June 28, Petty Officer Jeffrey Lucas, 33, was one of sixteen service members on board the Chinook helicopter downed by a rocket-propelled grenade during Operation Red Wings. He is survived by his widow, Rhonda; their son, Seth; his mother, Pat; his father, Richard; and his brother, Jamie. Jeff was laid to rest at Arlington National Cemetery in Section 60, stone 8229 and was posthumously decorated with the Bronze Star with Valor and the Purple Heart.

The Jeff Lucas Memorial Golf Tournament is now held annually to help raise funds for Corbett schools and scholarships awarded in Jeff's name; to make a contribution or to sign up for the event, please visit www.JeffLucasMemorial.com.

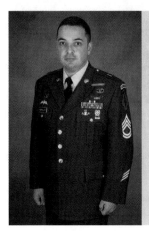

SERGEANT FIRST CLASS MARCUS MURALLES

Photo Credit: Arlingtoncemetery.com

Marcus grew up in Shelbyville, Indiana, and started active duty with the Army in 1989. He qualified as a medical specialist and served with Company B, 3rd Battalion, 75th Ranger Regiment at Fort Benning, Georgia until his initial commitment ended in 1993. After five years in the Army's reserve component, Marcus returned to active duty with 3rd Battalion and worked as a medical administrator and platoon medic. He relocated to Hunter Army Airfield, Georgia in 2003 with orders to 3rd Battalion, 160th Special Operations Aviation Regiment (Airborne). Marcus had already completed multiple deployments in the Middle East and returned to Afghanistan with the 160th in 2005.

On June 28, Sergeant First Class Marcus Muralles, 33, was serving on board the ill-fated Chinook as the flight medic. He is survived by his widow, Diana; their children, Anna and Dominic; his mother and stepfather, Rosemarie and Robert Dill; his father and stepmother, Leonel and Aura Muralles; his sister, Cindy; and his stepsister, Rhonda. Marcus was interred at Arlington National Cemetery in Section 60, stone 8199, and posthumously received the Bronze Star, the Purple Heart, and several other awards.

Marcus became an accomplished paratrooper and medic during his time in service; in addition, he earned his Ranger tab and was awarded jump qualifications from the British and German militaries. In 2006, 3rd Battalion dedicated the SFC Marcus V. Muralles Aid Station at Hunter Army Airfield in honor of Marcus and his devoted service.

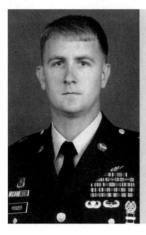

MASTER SERGEANT JAMES PONDER III

Photo Credit: Veterantributes.com

James "Tre" Ponder was a graduate of Battle Ground Academy in his hometown of Franklin, Tennessee. In 1990, he left Auburn University to enlist in the Army and completed training as a Chinook helicopter repairer. Tre was first assigned to Camp Humphries in Korea and worked there for two years as crew chief. He next reported to 2nd Battalion, 160th Special Operation Aviation Regiment (Airborne) based in Fort Campbell, Kentucky, where he spent the remainder of his time in the military. Tre served in a number of roles while stationed with the unit, to include platoon sergeant, team leader, flight commander, and instructor.

Tre conducted over 100 Special Operations missions during his career, and the deployment in 2005 was his fourth to Afghanistan. When the call went out on June 28 for a rescue mission to retrieve the entrenched SEALs, Tre knew he was more rested than the off-coming night crew and volunteered to go. Master Sergeant James Ponder III, 36, was on board the Chinook when it was shot down by enemy fire. He is survived by his widow, Leslie; his daughters, Samantha and Elizabeth; and his parents, Jimmy and Rebecca.

Tre was awarded a number of honors after his death, including the Bronze Star, the Purple Heart, and the Air Medal with Valor. He was also inducted into the Army Aviation Association of America's Hall of Fame in March 2015. To honor his memory, Tre's family started the Snowball Express 5k to benefit the children of fallen service members; visit their website at www.SnowballExpress5k.org.

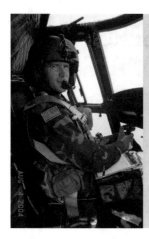

MAJOR STEPHEN REICH

Photo Credit: FOX Sports

Steve was brought up in Washington, Connecticut and graduated from the United States Military Academy at West Point in 1993. After receiving his commission in the Army, Steve reported to Fort Rucker, Alabama to complete basic aviation training and was designated an Army Aviator in March 1995. After serving in support of Operation Allied Force, Steve then received orders to the 160th Special Operations Aviation Regiment (Airborne) and deployed to Afghanistan with 2nd Battalion in 2001. He commanded Headquarters and Headquarters Company, 2nd Battalion from February 2002 through May 2003. Shortly after returning to the States, Steve assumed command of Company B, 3rd Battalion at Hunter Army Airfield, Georgia and prepared to return to Afghanistan.

Major Stephen Reich, 34, was serving as mission commander on board the lead Chinook when it was downed by a rocket-propelled grenade on June 28, 2005. He is survived by his widow, Jill; his parents, Ray and Sue; and his sisters, Megan and AnnMarie. Steve received a number of awards posthumously, including the Bronze Star, the Purple Heart, and the Meritorious Service Medal.

Shepaug Valley High School presents the Major Stephen Reich Memorial Award annually to a student who best exemplifies character, service, leadership, and achievement; with the award, the recipient is granted a sum of money to donate to the charity of their choice. For more information, please visit www.MajorReichAward.com.

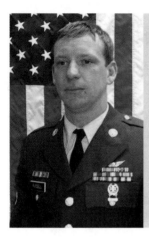

SERGEANT FIRST CLASS MICHAEL RUSSELL

Photo Credit: Gazingattheflag

Mike grew up playing baseball and football in the city of Stafford, Virginia. He enlisted in the Army after graduating from North Stafford High School in 1991 and completed training as a Chinook helicopter repairer. For the next three years, Mike served as a crew chief and flight engineer with Company B, 214th Aviation Regiment, 524th Corps Support Battalion at Schofield Barracks in Hawaii. He was then assigned to Company A, 2nd Battalion, 158th Aviation Regiment at Fort Carson in Colorado, and worked for the unit as a flight engineer. In 1996, Mike received his final orders to the 160th Special Operation Aviation Regiment (Airborne) and relocated to Hunter Army Airfield in Georgia.

During his time in service, Mike completed nine deployments to the Middle East. He had a reputation as a confident flight engineer who always went above and beyond the call of duty. Mike was also a devoted father, who spent all the time he could with his two daughters.

On June 28, 2005, Sergeant First Class Michael Russell, 31, was serving on the Chinook's flight crew when it was shot down by enemy fire. He is survived by his widow, Annette; their daughters, Lauren and Megan; his parents, Lee and Linda; and his siblings, Melissa and Lee. Mike received a number of decorations posthumously, including the Bronze Star, the Purple Heart, and the Air Medal with Valor.

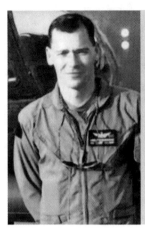

CHIEF WARRANT OFFICER 4 CHRIS SCHERKENBACH

Photo Credit: Foxsports.com

Chris grew up in the Mount Prospect neighborhood of Chicago, and graduated high school in 1982. He continued his education at Embry-Riddle Aeronautical University and completed his degree in professional aeronautics with distinction. In 1987, Chris enlisted in the Army as a communications specialist; he served for two years with the 270th Signal Company in West Germany before being accepted into the Warrant Officer program. Chris then attended Rotary Wing Aviator Training at Fort Rucker in Alabama and was designated an Army Aviator in 1991. His father had served in World War II as a bomber in the Army Air Force, and attended Chris' flight school graduation to pin on his wings.

After finishing his Chinook helicopter qualifications, Chris was stationed with Company B, 2nd Battalion, 159th Aviation Regiment at Hunter Army Airfield. He spent a year serving overseas in Korea, but returned to fly with the 159th until transferring to Company B, 3rd Battalion, 160th Special Operations Aviation Regiment (Airborne) in 1998.

On June 28, 2005, Chief Warrant Officer 4 Chris Scherkenbach, 40, was serving as a pilot on board the ill-fated Chinook. He is survived by his widow, Michelle; their daughter, Sarah Grace; his parents, Elmer and Marjorie; and his siblings, Jeff, Craig, Jed, Kurt, Lee, Karen, and Cheryl. For his service, Chris was posthumously decorated with a number of awards, including the Bronze Star, Purple Heart, and Master Army Aviator Badge. He was laid to rest in Arlington National Cemetery at Section 60, stone 8200.

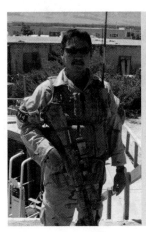

PETTY OFFICER SECOND CLASS JAMES SUH

Photo Credit: Mattaxelson.com

James was raised in Deerfield Beach, Florida. At the University of Florida, he began training during his freshman year to become a SEAL. James left for Navy boot camp in January 2001 and was originally trained as a quartermaster. He then entered Basic Underwater Demolition/SEAL training, and quickly earned a reputation for being prepared, dependable, and quiet with a wickedly dry sense of humor. After completing his advanced training, James was stationed with SEAL Delivery Vehicle Team ONE in Pearl Harbor.

The deployment to Afghanistan in 2005 would be James' first. When a rescue effort was coordinated on June 28, he was eager to go; his BUD/S classmate and friend, Matthew Axelson, was one of the men on the ground. Petty Officer Second Class James Suh, 28, was on board the Chinook when it was brought down by enemy fire. He is survived by his father, Solomon; and his sister, Claudia. James was posthumously awarded the Bronze Star with Valor and the Purple Heart.

At the Cupertino Veterans Memorial in California, a bronze sculpture called "The Guardians" depicts James and Matt crouching back-to-back, forever at the ready. Donations to the Memorial Park can be made at www.CupertinoVeteransMemorial.org. Additionally, the James Suh Memorial Scholarship is awarded to the student at Deerfield Beach High School who best reflects James' character. Contributions to the scholarship can be mailed to: The Exchange Club of Pompano Beach, Attn: James Suh Memorial Scholarship, P.O. Box 672, Pompano Beach, FL 33061.

PETTY OFFICER SECOND CLASS DANNY DIETZ

Danny was part of the SEAL team inserted into the Hindu Kush Mountains during Operation Red Wings. He was honored with the memorial workout on page 120.

CHIEF PETTY OFFICER JACQUES FONTAN

Jacques was one of the SEALs in the Quick Reaction Force on board the Chinook. He was memorialized with the workout on page 122.

LIEUTENANT MICHAEL MCGREEVY JR.

Mike was one of the SEALs on board the Chinook helicopter that was sent to rescue the reconnaissance team in the mountains. The workout dedicated to his memory can be found on page 124.

LIEUTENANT MICHAEL MURPHY

During Operation Red Wings, Michael was leading the four-man SEAL team on the ground. He is honored with the workout found on page 126.

PETTY OFFICER SECOND CLASS SHANE PATTON

Shane was a SEAL and was part of the rescue team on board the Chinook when it was shot down by enemy fire. The workout dedicated to his memory can be found on page 128.

PETTY OFFICER FIRST CLASS JEFFREY TAYLOR

Jeff was one of the SEALs on board the Chinook helicopter during Operation Red Wings. The workout dedicated to him can be found on page 132.

"The brave die never, though they sleep in dust:
their courage nerves a thousand living men."

Minot Judson Savage

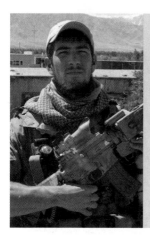

PETTY OFFICER SECOND CLASS DANNY DIETZ JR.

June 28, 2005

Photo Credit: Wikipedia.org

Danny was raised in Littleton, Colorado. He enlisted in the Navy in 1999 as a gunner's mate and entered Basic Underwater Demolition/SEAL training the following year. After finishing his advanced qualifications, Danny reported to SEAL Delivery Vehicle Team TWO in Little Creek, Virginia. His first deployment in April 2005 would take him to Afghanistan to support Operation Enduring Freedom.

During the night of June 27, Danny and three of his teammates left for a reconnaissance mission dubbed Operation Red Wings, and were dropped into enemy-controlled territory. Their position was compromised the next morning and the SEALs became engaged in a vicious firefight with an anti-coalition militia. Danny fought valiantly, continuing to fire at the enemy even after he lost a thumb and was shot multiple times. Petty Officer Second Class Danny Dietz, 25, was killed in action when another bullet struck his head. He is survived by his widow, Patsy; his parents, Dan Sr. and Cindy; and his siblings, Tiffany and Eric. For his extraordinary heroism in battle, Danny was posthumously awarded the Navy Cross. More information on Operation Red Wings can be found on page 102.

Danny's parents decided to share his story, and with the help of author Jer Dunlap, published *Danny: The Virtues Within* in 2014. Two charity organizations were also started in Danny's name: the Danny Dietz Memorial Scholarship Fund and The Danny Dietz Leadership & Training Foundation. Please visit www.NavySEALDannyDietz.com and www.Danny Dietz.org to make a contribution or to learn more about their programs.

DIETZ

10 rounds for time:
RUN (200M)
5 PULL-UPS
10 KB SWINGS (53/35LBS)
15 PUSH-UPS

Courtesy of Front Range CrossFit
Denver, Colorado

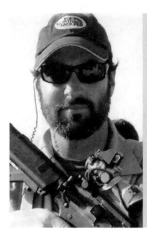

CHIEF PETTY OFFICER JACQUES FONTAN
June 28, 2005

Photo Credit: Pritzkermilitary.com

Jacques was raised in New Orleans, where he graduated from Brother Martin High School in 1986. While taking classes at the University of Louisiana, Jacques decided to enlist in the Navy. He was initially trained as a fire controlman and served aboard the USS Nicholas (FFG 47) until 1995. Jacques was then stationed with Helicopter Anti-Submarine Squadron ONE in Jacksonville, Florida to work as a rescue swimmer instructor. After nine years of service, he was selected to attend Basic Underwater Demolition/SEAL training and finished the course in 1998. Jacques would go on to work with SEAL Team EIGHT and Naval Special Warfare Group TWO, and completed deployments to Kosovo, Southeast Asia, and the Persian Gulf. In 2001, he reported to SEAL Team TEN and would later deploy with them to Afghanistan.

Chief Petty Officer Jacques Fontan, 36, was one of eight SEALs on board a Chinook helicopter when it was shot down by a rocket-propelled grenade. He is survived by his widow, Char Fontan Westfall; his daughter, Jourdan; his mother and stepfather, Hazel and Donald Rue; his father, Earl Fontan; and his siblings, Suzanne, Cheri, and Jean. Although he was originally buried in Jacksonville, Jacques was re-interred at Arlington National Cemetery, Section 60, stone 9752.

CrossFit Ferrum hosts Jacques' workout annually to raise funds for charity; they most recently made a contribution to All In, All The Time, a memorial foundation dedicated to helping Naval Special Warfare service members and their families. To learn more, go to www.AIATT.org.

FONTAN

For time:

36 BURPEES

Then, for 11 rounds:

11 FRONT SQUATS (115/75LBS)

11 PUSH PRESS (115/75LBS)

11 OVERHEAD SQUATS (115/75LBS)

36 BURPEES

Courtesy of CrossFit Ferrum
St. Johns, Florida

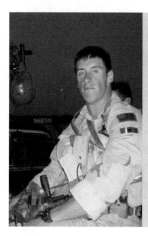

LIEUTENANT MICHAEL MCGREEVY JR.
June 28, 2005

Photo Credit: Laura McGreevy

Mike spent his high school years in Portville, New York. He set his sights on an appointment to the United States Naval Academy, holding out even after he was accepted early to West Point. In 1997, Mike commissioned as a surface warfare officer and served aboard the USS Oak Hill (LSD-51) until he was granted a lateral transfer to Special Warfare two years later. Mike went to complete deployments to South America and the Horn of Africa with SEAL Teams FOUR and Eight. He received orders to SEAL Team TEN in April 2004, and deployed to Afghanistan as the officer in charge of Echo Platoon the following year.

On June 28, 2005, Lieutenant Michael McGreevy, 30, was part of a Quick Reaction Force sent to help four entrenched SEALs during Operation Red Wings; he was on board an MH-47 Chinook helicopter when it was hit by enemy fire in Afghanistan. Mike is survived by his widow, Laura; their daughter, Molly; his mother, Patricia Mackin; and his father, Michael McGreevy, Sr. He was posthumously awarded the Bronze Star with Valor and the Purple Heart, and was laid to rest at Arlington National Cemetery in Section 60, stone 8230. To read more about the fateful events of Operation Red Wings, please see page 102.

In Portville, the McGreevy Memorial Run is held annually to benefit the Mike McGreevy Memorial Scholarship Fund. Scholarships are awarded in Mike's name to students in Portville and Virginia Beach who demonstrate integrity, humility, kindness, determination, and perseverance. Please visit their website at www.McGreevyRun.org.

MICHAEL

3 rounds for time:

RUN (800M)

50 BACK EXTENSIONS

50 SIT-UPS

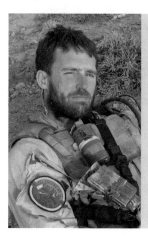

LIEUTENANT MICHAEL MURPHY
June 28, 2005

Photo Credit: Navy.mil

Michael was raised on Long Island, and graduated from Pennsylvania State University with degrees in political science and psychology. He commissioned through the Navy's Officer Candidate School in 2000 and entered Basic Underwater Demolition/SEAL training the following year. Michael then reported to SEAL Delivery Vehicle Team ONE in Pearl Harbor, Hawaii. He would go on to serve overseas in Jordan, Iraq, Qatar, and Djibouti, and left for a deployment to Afghanistan in 2005.

On the night of June 27, Michael led a four-man reconnaissance team through the mountains of Afghanistan on a mission dubbed Operation Red Wings. Their position was compromised the next morning and a battle with Taliban fighters ensued. Lieutenant Michael Murphy, 29, knowingly exposed himself to enemy fire in order to transmit a call to the Quick Reaction Force at Bagram Air Base; in risking his life for those of his teammates, Michael was shot and killed.

Michael is survived by his mother, Maureen; his father, Daniel; his brother, John; and his fiancée, Heather Duggan. In 2007, President Bush presented Michael's parents with his Medal of Honor; he was the first recipient of the medal for heroism in Afghanistan, and the first Navy recipient since the Vietnam War.

Michael's family now maintains the Lt. Michael P. Murphy Memorial Scholarship Foundation; the foundation is funded through donations and the annual Murph Challenge. To make a contribution or to sign up, please visit www.Murph Foundation.com and www.theMurphChallenge.com.

MURPH

For time, with optional 20-lb vest; partition pull-ups, push-ups, and squats as needed:

RUN (1 MILE)

100 PULL-UPS

200 PUSH-UPS

300 SQUATS

RUN (1 MILE)

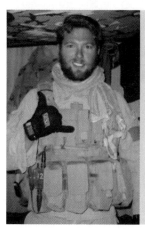

PETTY OFFICER SECOND CLASS SHANE PATTON

June 28, 2005

Photo Credit: Findagrave.com

Shane was born in San Diego, California and moved to Boulder City, Nevada at the age of eleven. He grew up surfing and skateboarding, and stood out as the star pitcher and outfielders on the baseball team at Boulder City High School. Shane chose to follow after his father, a former Navy SEAL, and enlisted in the Navy in 2000. He entered Basic Underwater Demolition/SEAL training the following year and completed several advanced skills courses before reporting to SEAL Delivery Vehicle Team ONE in Pearl Harbor, Hawaii.

Shane deployed with his team to Afghanistan in April 2005. On 28 June, he was part of a rescue effort sent to recover the four SEALs who had come under enemy fire during Operation Red Wings. Petty Officer Second Class Shane Patton, 22, was on board a Chinook helicopter when it was shot down by a rocket-propelled grenade. He is survived by his father and stepmother, James and Pamela Patton; his mother, Valerie Berdeski; and his brothers, James II, Chase, and Dean. Shane was posthumously decorated with the Bronze Star with Valor and the Purple Heart, and was laid to rest with full military honors in his hometown. To read more about Operation Red Wings, please go to page 102.

Shane's friends started a scholarship in his name to benefit students of Boulder City High School, and host a memorial pub crawl to help raise funds. For more information on making donations, please e-mail thedillingergroup@gmail.com.

SHANE

For time:

25 DEADLIFTS (155/105lbs)

RUN (400M)

10 PULL-UPS*

10 GROUND-TO-OVERHEADS (155/105lbs)

RUN (800M)

10 PULL-UPS

[Continued on next page]

[Continued from previous page]

10 GROUND-TO-OVERHEADS (155/105lbs)

10 PULL-UPS

RUN (800M)

10 GROUND-TO-OVERHEADS (155/105lbs)

10 PULL-UPS

RUN (400M)

25 DEADLIFTS (155/105lbs)

Workout Notes
*Strict pull-ups

Courtesy of SinCity CrossFit
Henderson, Nevada

"War is an ugly thing, but not the ugliest of things: the decayed and degraded state of moral and patriotic feeling which thinks that nothing is worth a war, is much worse…A man who has nothing which he is willing to fight for, nothing which he cares more about than he does about his personal safety, is a miserable creature who has no chance of being free, unless made and kept so by the exertions of better men than himself."

John Stuart Mill

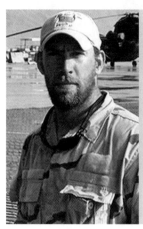

PETTY OFFICER FIRST CLASS JEFFREY TAYLOR
June 28, 2005

Photo Credit: Veteranstributes.com

Jeff grew up in Hotchkiss, West Virginia and left for Navy boot camp in 1994. He spent five years serving as a hospital corpsman before entering the SEAL training pipeline, and was first stationed with SEAL Team EIGHT. He later worked aboard the USS Theodore Roosevelt (CVN-71) and at the John F. Kennedy Special Warfare Center at Fort Bragg, but received his final set of orders to SEAL Team TEN. In April 2005, Jeff deployed to Afghanistan as his platoon's leading petty officer.

A rescue effort was launched to recover four SEALs who had come under attack during Operation Red Wings on June 28, 2005. Petty Officer First Class Jeffrey Taylor, 30, was on board the Chinook helicopter when it was hit by enemy fire. He is survived by his widow, Erin; his mother and stepfather, Gail and John Bowman; his father and stepmother, John and Cheryl Taylor; his brother, Brandon Cox; his half-brothers, Justin and Josh Taylor; and his stepbrothers, James, Jay, Kelly, and Carl Bowman. Jeff was posthumously awarded the Bronze Star with Valor and the Purple Heart, and a marker bearing his name can be found at Arlington National Cemetery in Memorial Section F, stone 25-5. To read more about the story of Operation Red Wings, please go to page 102.

In lieu of flowers at his funeral, Jeff's family requested donations be made in his name to the Navy SEAL Foundation. Since 2000, they have provided support to Naval Special Warfare service members and their families. Visit them at www.NavySealFoundation.org.

JT

For time, 21/15/9 reps in circuit:

HANDSTAND PUSH-UPS

RING DIPS

PUSH-UPS

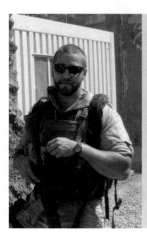

PETTY OFFICER FIRST CLASS JASON LEWIS
July 6, 2007

Photo Credit: News.crossfitdauntless.com.au

Jason was raised in Brookfield, Connecticut. After graduating high school, he began taking classes at the University of Maryland. Jason spent a year in college before enlisting in the in Navy, and finished Basic Underwater Demolition/SEAL training in August 1997. He then completed the Basic Airborne Course at Fort Benning, Georgia, Jason and was assigned to SEAL Team FIVE in Coronado, California until March 2004. Jason then worked at the Naval Special Warfare Center for nearly two years and, in 2006, received orders to an East Coast-based SEAL Team.

On July 6, Petty Officer First Class Jason Lewis, 30, was deployed to Iraq and working near Baghdad. He and his teammates were returning from an operation when a homemade bomb detonated under his Humvee; the blast took his life and those of two other Sailors. Jason is survived by his widow, Donna; their three children, Jack, Max, and Grace; his mother, Jean Mariano; his father, Dale Lewis; and his sister, Jennie Schell. He was buried near his hometown with full military honors, and posthumously awarded the Bronze Star with Valor and the Purple Heart.

In lieu of flowers at his memorial, Jason's family requested donations be made in his name to the Navy SEAL Foundation. Please visit their website at www.NavySEALFoundation.org to make a contribution. Jason's widow, Donna, has also participated in several empowerment events hosted by the Travis Manion Foundation, including a swim across the English Channel. To learn more about the mission of TMF, please visit www.TravisManion.org.

JASON

For time:

**100 SQUATS
5 MUSCLE-UPS**

**75 SQUATS
10 MUSCLE-UPS**

**50 SQUATS
15 MUSCLE-UPS**

**25 SQUATS
20 MUSCLE-UPS**

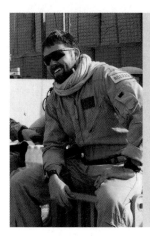

SERGEANT MICHAEL ROY
July 8, 2009

Photo Credit: Patriotcrossfit.com

Michael spent the beginning of his childhood in Candia, New Hampshire and later moved to North Fort Myers, Florida. He was committed to joining the military from a young age, and enlisted in the Marine Corps after the terror attacks of 9/11. Michael trained as a rifleman and, over the next few years, completed multiple tours of duty overseas in Japan, Haiti, and Iraq. In March 2008, he joined Marine Corps Forces Special Operations and reported to 3rd Marine Special Operations Battalion at Camp Lejeune, North Carolina. Michael left on his third deployment to the Middle East before the birth of his youngest child, but was granted leave to visit his family and meet his son. He went back to Afghanistan, scheduled to return home only a few weeks later.

On July 8, 2009, Sergeant Michael Roy, 25, was shot by an enemy sniper during combat operations in the Nimroz province. He is survived by his widow, Amy; their children, Michael, Olivia, and Landon; his mother, Lisa Hickey; his father, Michael Roy; and his siblings, Richard, Joshua, and Christine. In honor of his dedicated service, Michael was posthumously decorated with the Bronze Star and the Purple Heart.

The MARSOC Foundation was established to assist active duty and medically retired MARSOC personnel and their families in times of need; they also provide financial aid and support services to the families of fallen MARSOC Marines and Sailors. To make a donation in Michael's name, please visit www.MARSOC Foundation.org.

ROY

5 rounds for time:

15 DEADLIFTS (225lbs)

20 BOX JUMPS (24")

25 PULL-UPS

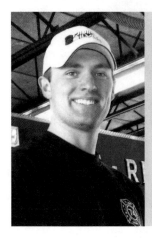

FIREFIGHTER RYAN HUMMERT
July 21, 2008

Photo Credit: Crossfit

Ryan grew up just west of St. Louis in Maplewood, Missouri. He excelled academically at Rockwood Summit High School and was awarded a football scholarship to play at Missouri Valley College. Ryan's athletic career was cut short by a knee injury, and he chose to instead pursue a career in the fire department. After completing paramedic training in 2007, Ryan was hired by the Maplewood Fire Department and graduated from the St. Louis County Fire Academy the following March. During his short time with the department, Ryan was credited with saving someone's life when he resuscitated them after a heart attack.

Ryan's team answered the call for a vehicle fire early on the morning of July 21, 2008—Ryan's first official fire response. Shortly after the crew arrived on scene, Firefighter Ryan Hummert, 22, was shot and killed by a sniper. The man had positioned himself in a house across the street and lit the fire to attract emergency responders; he shot Ryan and two police officers before ending his own life. Ryan is survived by his parents, Andy and Jackie; and his sister, Ashley.

The City of Maplewood rededicated a local park as the Ryan Hummert Memorial Park, and commissioned a sculpture of Ryan in his turnout gear. The city also maintains a scholarship in his honor, which is awarded to Emergency Medical Technicians working toward their paramedic certification. To make a donation or to read more, please visit the "Fire Department" page at www.CityOf Maplewood.com.

RYAN

5 rounds for time:

7 MUSCLE-UPS

21 BURPEES

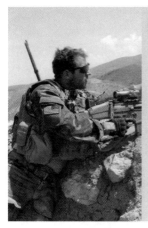

SERGEANT
JUSTIN HANSEN
July 24, 2012

Photo Credit: Frank Parisi

Justin was a native of Kingsley, Michigan and graduated high school in 2003. After several semesters at Northwestern Michigan College, he chose to enlist in the Marine Corps and completed the School of Infantry. Justin was then selected for Basic Reconnaissance Course, followed by orders to 3rd Reconnaissance Battalion at Camp Schwab in Okinawa, Japan. He later deployed to the Middle East with the 31st Marine Expeditionary Unit and, in 2009, Justin reported to 2nd Marine Special Operations Battalion at Camp Lejeune, North Carolina, and soon began preparing for this third deployment to the Middle East.

On July 24, 2012, Sergeant Justin Hansen, 26, was on a raid in the Badghis province of Afghanistan when he was mortally wounded by enemy fire. His partner, Staff Sergeant Andrew Seif, completed their objective and rendered medical aid but Justin succumbed to his wounds. He leaves behind his mother and stepfather, Vickie Hays and Steven Cornell; his father and stepmother, Richard and Shawna Hansen; his sisters Adrienne, Morgan, and Veronica; and his stepsiblings, Jeremy, Adam, and Jessica. In honor of his dedicated service, the Marine Corps posthumously awarded Justin the Bronze Star with Valor and the Purple Heart.

Kingsley High School paid tribute to Justin by retiring his jersey, no. 54, in a ceremony shortly after his death. Please consider making a donation in his name to the MARSOC Foundation, which provides support to Special Operations Marines and their families. Visit their website at www.MARSOCFoundation.org.

JUSTIN

For time, 30/20/10 reps in circuit:

BACK SQUATS*

BENCH PRESSES*

PULL-UPS**

Workout Notes
*Lbs equal to bodyweight
**Strict pull-ups

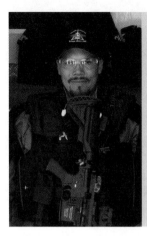

DETECTIVE CARLOS LEDESMA
July 28, 2010

Photo Credit: Eastvalleycrossfit.com

Carlos grew up in Stockton, California. While attending Amos Alonzo Stagg High School, he turned down a college music scholarship to enlist in the Marine Corps after graduation. Carlos spent eight years on active duty and became a veteran of the Persian Gulf War. After leaving the military, he completed his associate's degree in criminal justice and first served as a patrol officer in the small town of Spirit Lake, Iowa.

In 2007, Carlos joined the police department in Chandler, Arizona; he became a detective and started working undercover in narcotics. On the evening of July 28, 2010, Carlos and two other officers were participating in a drug sting involving hundreds of pounds of marijuana and a quarter million dollars. Detective Carlos Ledesma, 34, died in the line of duty when he was shot four times in the chest; the other two officers were injured in the ensuing shoot out. Though the death penalty was originally sought for Carlos' killer, prosecution and sentencing was still ongoing in 2016. Carlos is survived by his widow and their two sons; his parents, Reynaldo and Dora Rae; and his sister, Trina Ledesma-Leung.

Amos Alonzo Stagg High School grants two annual scholarships in Carlos' honor to senior athletes or band members; for more information, contact the school via www.ASHS-SUSD-CA.SchoolLoop.com. Please consider a donation in Carlos' name to the 100 Club of Arizona, an organization dedicated to supporting first responders and their families; visit them at www.100Club.org.

LEDESMA

In 20 minutes, as many rounds as possible:

5 PARALLETTE HANDSTAND PUSH-UPS

10 TOES-THROUGH-RINGS

15 MEDICINE BALL CLEANS (20lbs)

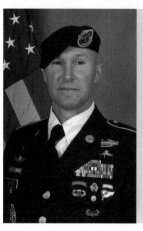

SERGEANT FIRST CLASS SEVERIN SUMMERS III

August 2, 2009

Photo Credit: Sincitycrossfit.com

Sev was born in Lafayette, Louisiana. After graduating from Louisiana State University, he enlisted in the Army National Guard as an infantryman in 1989. Sev completed the Special Forces Qualification Course to earn his Green Beret in 2002 and was assigned to 2nd Battalion, 20th Special Forces Group (Airborne). He later finished Ranger School and joined Operational Detachment-Alpha 2065, the SCUBA team.

In 2009, Sec volunteered to leave job as a recruiter to mobilize with Company C, 2nd Battalion, 20th Special Forces Group (Airborne). It was his second tour of duty in Afghanistan and, as an engineer sergeant, he was responsible for both construction and demolition in his unit. On August 2, 2009, Sergeant First Class Severin Summers, 43, was killed on a combat patrol near Qole Gerdsar when his vehicle was hit by an improvised explosive device. He is survived by his widow, Tammy; his daughters, Shelby, Jessica, and Sarah; his parents, West and Charlene; his brothers, Sean, Pierre, and William; and his sister, Andree. Sev's body was escorted home by his brother, Captain Sean Summers, and laid to rest at Arlington National Cemetery in Section 60, stone 8653. For his dedicated service, Sev was posthumously awarded the Bronze Star and the Purple Heart.

Sev's family requested donations in his name be made to Patriots and Heroes Outdoors. Formerly called Hunts for Heroes, the organization facilitates recreational experiences like hunting and fishing for injured veterans and their families. Please visit them at www.PatriotsAndHeroes Outdoors.com to make a contribution.

SEVERIN

For time, with optional 20-lb vest:

50 PULL-UPS*

100 PUSH-UPS**

RUN (5 KM)

Workout Notes
*Strict pull-ups
**Hand release

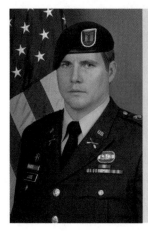

CAPTAIN RONALD LUCE JR.
August 2, 2009

Photo Credit: Arlingtoncemetery.net

Ron was raised in Julian, California. As a cadet at the Valley Forge Military Academy in Wayne, Pennsylvania, he commissioned in the Army National Guard in 2002 and then completed his biology degree at Belmont University in Nashville. Ron earned a number of military qualifications, finishing Ranger School, the Basic Airborne Course, and the Special Forces Qualification Course. After earning his Green Beret in 2008, Ron initially served as a liaison officer with 2nd Battalion, 7th Special Forces Group (Airborne), but was reassigned to Company C, 2nd Battalion, 20th Special Forces Group (Airborne) to serve as a detachment commander.

On August 2, 2009, Captain Ronald Luce, 27, was killed during a combat patrol in Afghanistan when his vehicle hit an improvised explosive device; the blast also took the lives of two other Soldiers. Ron is survived by his widow, Kendahl; his daughter, Carrie; his parents, Ronald Sr. and Katherine; and his nine brothers and sisters. For his dedicated service, Ron was posthumously decorated with the Bronze Star and the Purple Heart; he was laid to rest in Arlington National Cemetery in Section 60, stone 8946.

In 2015, Ron's family participated in the Army Ten Miler to raise funds for the Tragedy Assistance Program for Survivors. The program been dedicated to families suffering from the loss of a service member since 1994, and provides access to a nationwide peer-support and resource network at no cost to the family. Please consider visiting their website, www.TAPS.org, to make a contribution in memory of Ron.

LUCE

3 rounds for time, with 20-lb vest:

RUN (1 KM)

10 MUSCLE-UPS

100 SQUATS

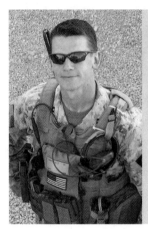

CAPTAIN
GARRETT LAWTON
August 4, 2008

Photo Credit: Iraqwarheroes.org

Garrett was first photographed in a Marine Corps uniform when he was eight years old. In 1999, he completed degrees in mechanical and aerospace engineering at West Virginia University and commissioned in the Marines Corps as a flight officer. Garrett trained as an F/A-18D Hornet Weapons System Operator and reported to Marine All-Weather Fighter Attack Squadron 244 at Marine Corps Air Station Beaufort, South Carolina. He completed a deployment to Iraq in 2005 and was subsequently selected to serve with Marine Corps Forces Special Operations. Garrett reported to the 2nd Marine Special Operations Battalion in Camp Lejeune and was sent to Afghanistan in 2008.

Garrett's convoy was attacked on May 29, and he sustained injuries while trying to save a Soldier trapped in a burning vehicle; he'd then refused medical evacuation and stayed on-site to coordinate air support and the prosecution of enemy targets. On August 4, 2008, Captain Garrett Lawton, 31, was mortally wounded when his vehicle was hit by the detonation of an improvised explosive device. He is survived by his widow, Trisha; his sons, Ryan and Caden; his mother and stepfather, Catherine and Cal Peters; his father, David Lawton; and his sister, Kenna Hubai.

Garrett was laid to rest at Arlington National Cemetery, Section 60, stone 8742 and posthumously decorated with the Bronze Star with Valor and two Purple Hearts. His family requested that donations in his name be made to The Wounded Warrior Fund; for more information on their programs and initiatives, please visit www.WoundedWarriorProject.org.

GARRETT

3 rounds for time:
75 SQUATS
25 RING HANDSTAND PUSH-UPS
25 L PULL-UPS

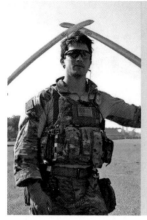

MASTER SERGEANT JARED VAN AALST
August 4, 2010

Photo Credit: Jvafoundation.org

Jared grew up in Laconia, New Hampshire and enlisted in the Army in 1995. Originally trained as signal support systems specialist, he completed the Basic Airborne Course and the Ranger Indoctrination Program. Jared then reported to Headquarters and Headquarters Company, 3rd Battalion, 75th Ranger Regiment and graduated from Ranger School during the summer of 1997. He retrained as a sniper the following year, and was later selected for instructor duty at the U.S. Army Marksmanship Unit. Jared returned to 3rd Battalion in 2003 and completed five tours of duty in Iraq and Afghanistan over the next five years. In 2008, he received orders to the Army Special Operations Command at Fort Bragg, North Carolina.

Master Sergeant Jared Van Aalst, 34, was mortally wounded during combat operations in the Kunduz province of Afghanistan on August 4, 2010. He is survived by his widow, Katie; his daughters, Kaylie and Ava; his parents, Neville and Nancy; and four siblings. Jared's son, Hugh Jared, was born after his death. In recognition of his service, Jared was posthumously awarded the Bronze Star with Valor and the Purple Heart, and was laid to rest at Arlington National Cemetery in Section 60, stone 9259.

Jared was two months away from earning his bachelor's degree at the time of his death. In his honor, the MSG Jared Van Aalst Memorial Foundation awards four scholarships to students pursing higher education. Please visit www.JVAFoundation.org to sign up for a competitive event or to make a contribution.

JARED

4 rounds for time:

RUN (800M)

40 PULL-UPS

70 PUSH-UPS

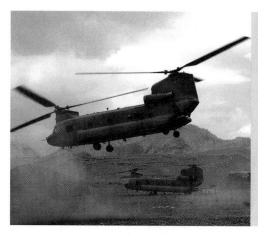

31 HEROES
August 6, 2011

Photo Credit: Wikipedia.org

On August 6, 2011, a CH-47D Chinook departed from a forward operating base south of Kabul, Afghanistan. On board the helicopter, call sign Extortion 17, was an Immediate Reaction Force consisting of five Army aviation crewmembers, three Air Force Special Operations personnel, 22 Naval Special Warfare personnel, one military working dog, and eight Afghans. They had been dispatched to support the 75th Ranger Regiment—the Rangers had secured an insurgent compound and were tracking down fleeing militants. As the Chinook made its approach to the designated landing zone, two enemy fighters ran out of a building and launched rocket-propelled grenades. The first round missed the helicopter, but the second struck its rear rotor blade. The resulting explosion severed a large section of the blade, causing a disastrous imbalance and tearing the Chinook apart. The helicopter spun out of control and crashed in a creek bed moments after being hit by the projectile. There were no survivors.

The loss of 31 military service members was devastating. In the wake of the tragedy, the 31 Heroes Project was founded to support the families affected by the crash of Extortion 17. Their memorial workout is hosted annually by hundreds of gyms across the country to honor the memories of the fallen and raise funds for the 31 Heroes Project. Since 2011, more than $1.5 million has been given back to military service members and their families through grant-making opportunities and partnership programs. To make a contribution or to sign up for the workout event, please visit www.31Heroes.com.

31HEROES

In 31 minutes, as many rounds as possible:

8 THRUSTERS (155/105lbs)

6 ROPE CLIMBS (15')

11 BOX JUMPS (30"/24")

Partner Option

Partner 1 performs the workout listed above while Partner 2 runs 400M while carrying a sand bag (45/25lbs). When Partner 2 returns from the run, Partner 1 will take the sandbag and begin their 400M run; Partner 2 will continue the workout where Partner 1 left off. Repeat for 31 minutes.

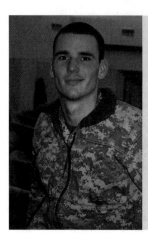

SERGEANT ALEXANDER BENNETT

Photo Credit: Stripes.com

Alex grew up in Tacoma, Washington, and he joined the Washington National Guard as a rifleman in 2004. Three years later, he enlisted in the U.S. Army Reserve and qualified as a Chinook helicopter repairer. Even more than he liked working on cars, Alex loved working on helicopters and was planning to make a career in the Army; he had aspirations to become a pilot one day. While stationed at Joint Base Lewis-McCord in Washington, Alex deployed to Iraq in 2009 with 1st Battalion, 214th Aviation Regiment. He requested a transfer to Company B, 158th Aviation Regiment in Gardner, Kansas knowing he would deploy again and have more opportunities to fly.

On August 6, 2011, Specialist Alexander Bennett, 24, was serving as a flight engineer on board the Chinook when it was shot down. He is survived by his mother, Kim Robertson, and his father, Douglas Bennett. Alex was laid to rest at Arlington National Cemetery in Section 60, stone 9942, and was posthumously promoted to the rank of Sergeant. He was additionally awarded the Bronze Star and the Purple Heart in recognition of his honorable service.

The Wounded Warrior Project was an organization that Alex proudly supported; his family requested that donations be made to them in his name. To make a contribution or to read more about their current initiatives, please visit www.WoundedWarriorProject.org.

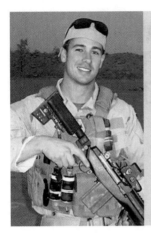

CHIEF PETTY OFFICER DARRIK BENSON

Photo Credit: Findagrave.com

Darrik grew up in the Napa Valley of California, in a small community called Angwin. He enlisted in the Navy at the age of 17 and left for boot camp after his graduation in 2001. Darrik initially qualified as an aviation ordnanceman, then entered Basic Underwater Demolition/SEAL training the following year. After reporting to SEAL Team THREE in 2003, he completed multiple deployments to support Operations Iraqi Freedom. Darrick then successfully screened for the Naval Special Warfare Development Group and relocated to the East Coast in 2009.

Both driven and kind, Darrick had a sharp focus that helped him achieve excellence in everything he attempted. He met the woman he intended to marry while stationed in San Diego, and together they had a son named Landon. From then on, Darrik always kept one of his son's toy airplanes in his pack when he deployed overseas, a small reminder of home. After leaving military service, he planned to use his pilot's license to fly commercially.

On August 6, 2011, Petty Officer First Class Darrik Benson, 28, was on board the Chinook when it crashed. He is survived by his fiancée, Kara Nakamura; their son, Landon; his mother, Beverly Nieman Mills; his father, Fred Benson; and his sister, Brianna Benson. In recognition of Darrik's sacrifice, he was posthumously promoted to the rank of Chief Petty Officer.

When recovery teams searched the wreckage of the Chinook, one of the few items they recovered was a toy airplane.

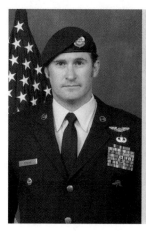

TECHNICAL SERGEANT JOHN BROWN

Photo Credit: Travismanion.org

John grew up in Siloam Springs, Arkansas. He attended John Brown University on a swimming scholarship and planned to become a nurse anesthetist. While taking pre-med courses, John saw a Special Operations video that changed the course of his life. He enlisted in the Air Force in 2002, and qualifying as Pararescueman. As a PJ, John would be responsible for rendering medical aid to those in need and extracting them from dangerous situations when necessary.

After more than two years of training, John was assigned to the 38th Rescue Squadron at Moody Air Force Base in Georgia. He worked with the unit until March 2006, then transferred overseas to the 31st Rescue Squadron at Kadena Air Force Base in Japan. John completed three additional years of service before he was accepted for a position with the 24th Special Tactics Squadron at Pope Air Force Base, North Carolina. During his career, he would serve multiple deployments in Iraq and Afghanistan to support Operations Iraqi Freedom and Enduring Freedom.

On August 6, 2011, Sergeant John Brown, 33, was killed when the helicopter he was on board was shot down by an enemy rocket-propelled grenade. He is survived by his widow, Tabitha; his father, Dan Brown; his mother, Elizabeth Newlun; and his brothers, Danny and Lucas. John was laid to rest at Arlington National Cemetery in Section 60, stone 9941, and was decorated with the Bronze Star. Having been recently selected for advancement in rank, John was posthumously promoted to Technical Sergeant.

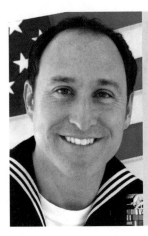

CHIEF PETTY OFFICER CHRISTOPHER CAMPBELL

Photo Credit: Arlingtoncemetery.net

The son of a Master Gunnery Sergeant, Chris grew up near Camp Lejeune in Jacksonville, North Carolina. He enlisted in the Navy in 1996 and entered Basic Underwater Demolition/SEAL training a year later. Chris was first stationed with SEAL Team FIVE, and later worked at a training detachment in Key West before receiving orders to the Naval Special Warfare Development Group. During his military service, Chris completed multiple combat deployments to Iraq and Afghanistan.

Petty Officer First Class Christopher Campbell, 36, was on board the Chinook when it was shot down on August 6, 2011. He is survived by his widow, Angelina; their daughter, Samantha; his parents, Larry and Diane; and his siblings, Le and Cindy. Chris was laid to rest in Arlington National Cemetery alongside many of his teammates in Section 60, stone 9929, and received a posthumous promotion to the rank of Chief Petty Officer.

In the event of his death, Chris requested that his hometown newspaper run a story on him for a good cause. He asked that the article direct donations to veteran aid organizations in the hopes that 100,000 people would send money. In honoring his final wish, please consider the Navy SEAL Foundation, an organization dedicated to helping Naval Special Warfare service members and their families. Visit them at www.NavySEALFoundation.org. Additionally, the Frogman 3D Bowhunters Challenge and 5k Trail Run is held in Jacksonville to remember Chris and to raise money for wounded veterans. For more information, please go their Facebook page.

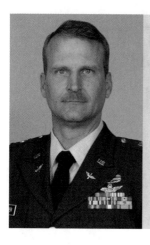

CHIEF WARRANT OFFICER 5 DAVID CARTER

Photo Credit: Veterantributes.com

Dave was raised in Hays, Kansas and enlisted in the U.S. Army Reserve in 1983. Two years later, he joined the Kansas Army National Guard and worked with the 435th General Support Aviation Company in Hutchinson as a petroleum-handling specialist. After completing his zoology degree at Fort Hays University in 1987, Dave was selected for the National Guard's Warrant Officer program. He then attended flight school and was designated a rotary wing aviator the following year.

Throughout his career, Dave piloted Iroquois, Kiowa, Cobra, and Chinook helicopters and became one of the National Guard's most accomplished instructor pilots. He had both the talent and temperament required for molding new pilots and served multiple stints on active duty. In 2005, Dave was assigned to 2nd Battalion, 135th Aviation Regiment at Buckley Air Force Base in Colorado, where he remained for the duration of his time in service. He deployed the following year to Iraq and logged over 700 hours of combat flight.

Chief Warrant Officer 4 David Carter, 47, deployed to Afghanistan in 2011 and was serving as one of the Chinook's pilots when it was downed by enemy fire on August 6. He is survived by his widow, Laura; their children, Kyle and Kaitlen; his mother, Elsie; his brothers, Bill, Mark, and Paul; and his half-brother, Paul. Dave was promoted posthumously to the rank of Chief Warrant Officer 5, and was decorated with the Legion of Merit Medal, the Bronze Star, and the Purple Heart.

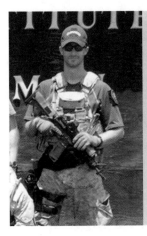

PETTY OFFICER FIRST CLASS JARED DAY

Photo Credit: Sandiegouniontribune.com // US Navy

Jared was born in Salt Lake City, and grew up in the nearby town of Taylorsville. He announced his plans to join the military at the age of six, and surrounded himself with military toys and games. After graduating from Cottonwood High School in 2001, Jared enlisted in the Navy and left for boot camp in November of the following year. He then qualified as an information systems technician, a job which made him responsible for a variety of computer and communications functions.

Jared spent a year serving at his first duty station, Naval Computer and Telecommunications Station Keflavik in Iceland, and was subsequently stationed at the Naval Special Warfare Command in Coronado, California. In 2007, he was selected for assignment to the Naval Special Warfare Development Group and worked to support SEAL team operations as a Tactical Communicator. During his time in service, Jared completed his Expeditionary Warfare and Free Fall Parachutist qualifications, and deployed to locations in Africa, Asia, and the Middle East.

Petty Officer First Class Jared Day, 28, lost his life in the Chinook crash on August 6, 2011. Along with Petty Officer First Class Michael Strange, Jared was posthumously awarded the National Intelligence Medal for Valor. He is survived by his mother, Karolyn Kimball Day; his father, Sam Day; and his sister, Geri.

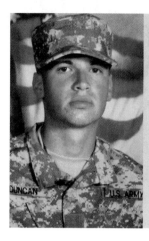

SPECIALIST SPENCER DUNCAN

Photo Credit: Travismanion.org

"Have a great day. Make it count." These were the words the Duncan brothers heard their father say every morning. Growing up in Olathe, Kansas, Spencer graduated from Olathe South High School in 2008. He knew he wanted to make a difference in the world, and chose to join the U.S. Army Reserve the following June. After basic training in Fort Knox, Kentucky, Spencer qualified as a helicopter repairer and was stationed near his hometown with 7th Battalion, 158th Aviation Regiment. He loved working as a mechanic and became a door gunner for Chinook helicopters. In May 2011, Spencer was sent to Afghanistan for his first deployment.

Specialist Spencer Duncan, 21, was a member of the Chinook's aircrew when it was shot down in the Wardak province on August 6, 2011. He is survived by his parents, Dale and Megan; his brothers, Tanner and Calder; and his beloved dog, Dixie. When Spencer's body was brought home to Olathe, 15,000 people turned out to line the roads and show solidarity with the Duncan family.

The Make It Count Foundation was started in honor of Spencer and the sacrifice he made while serving our country. The non-profit foundation makes contributions to a number of organizations that provide support to veterans, and hosts an annual 5k run to help raise funds. To make a contribution or to register for the race, please visit www.MakeIt CountToday.org.

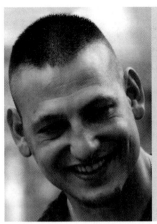

STAFF SERGEANT PATRICK HAMBURGER

Photo Credit: Army.togetherweserved.com

Patrick was raised in Lincoln, Nebraska. He enlisted in the Army National Guard in 1998 and left for basic training after graduating high school the following year. Initially qualified as a petroleum supply specialist, Patrick retrained as a helicopter repairer and was assigned to Troop F, 1st Battalion, 167th Air Calvary Squadron in his hometown. He had always enjoyed repairing cars, and quickly found that he loved maintaining the Cobra, Apache, and Kiowa helicopters for which he was responsible. In 2004, he began serving in Troop D of the same unit (now the 124th Air Calvary Squadron), and was introduced to Chinook helicopters. Patrick transferred two years later to Company B, 2nd Battalion, 135th Aviation Regiment, based in Grand Island and began working full-time as a flight engineer. In 2011, he was mobilized for deployment to Afghanistan.

Sergeant Patrick Hamburger, 30, was killed while serving as a member of the Chinook's aircrew when it was shot down by enemy fire on August 6. He is survived by his girlfriend, Candie Reagan; their daughters, Veronica and Payton; his mother and stepfather, Joyce and DeLayne Peck; his father and stepmother, Douglas and Shaune Hamburger; his brothers, Michael and Christopher Hamburger; and his stepsiblings, Jessica, Jeremy, and Joshua Francis. Patrick's body was accompanied home by Candie's brother, Sergeant David Mason. In recognition of his dedicated service, Patrick was posthumously promoted to Staff Sergeant, and awarded the Bronze Star and the Purple Heart.

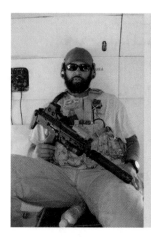

CHIEF PETTY OFFICER KEVIN HOUSTON

Photo Credit: Arlingtoncemetery.net

Kevin moved from San Jose, California to West Hyannisport, Massachusetts in the fifth grade; even then, he had already decided to become a Navy SEAL. But Kevin's road to Naval Special Warfare would be harder for him than many others: during his senior year in high school, he broke his back in a motorcycle accident.

Kevin graduated in 1994 and, in spite of his injury, enlisted in the Navy the following year. Initially trained as an aviation electrician's mate, he served with Strike Fighter Squadron 195 aboard the USS Independence (CV-62) and with Helicopter Anti-Submarine Squadron TWO in San Diego. Kevin began Basic Underwater Demolition/SEAL training in 1998 and was subsequently assigned to SEAL Team FOUR in Virginia Beach. He completed a deployment to Iraq in 2005, then spent two years as a weapons instructor at the Naval Special Warfare Group TWO training Detachment. In 2008, Kevin was assigned to the Naval Special Warfare Development Group and remained with the elite unite for the duration of his service.

On August 6, 2011, Chief Petty Officer Kevin Houston, 36, was on board the Chinook helicopter when it was brought down by enemy fire in Afghanistan. He is survived by his widow, Meiling; their children, Michael, Jaina, and Ethan; his mother, Jan Anderson; his brother, Craig; and his father, Arthur Houston. Kevin was laid to rest at Arlington National Cemetery in Section 60, stone 9931. To honor his memory, Barnstable High School retired his Red Raiders jersey, no. 46, in 2014.

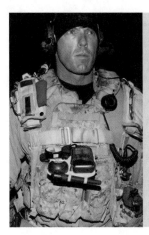

MASTER CHIEF PETTY OFFICER LOUIS LANGLAIS

Photo Credit: Veterantributes.com

Lou was born in Quebec, Canada, and moved to Santa Barbara, California, when he was nine. In June 1986, he enlisted in the Navy as a boatswain's mate and served on the USS Wadsworth (FFG-9). In February 1989, Lou began training as a SEAL. He spent seven years with SEAL Team THREE and, during the Persian Gulf War, deployed to Southwest Asia to support Operations Desert Shield and Desert Storm. Lou was next assigned to the "The Leap Frogs," the Navy's precision parachute team, and made the national news in 1997: while attempting to jump into the Florida Marlin's stadium dressed as their mascot, high winds detached the head of his costume. Lou landed safely in a parking lot, and Billy the Marlin's head was later found near the Florida Turnpike.

In 2000, Lou was selected to serve with the Naval Special Warfare Development Group. He relocated to Virginia Beach and went on to complete multiple tours of duty overseas in Iraq and Afghanistan. With almost 25 years on active duty, Lou was slated to become a trainer for other SEALs after returning from his upcoming deployment.

On August 6, 2011, Master Chief Petty Officer Louis Langlais, 44, was on board the Chinook when it was shot down by a rocket-propelled grenade in Afghanistan. He is survived by his widow, Anya; their sons, Gabe and Jack; and his siblings, Jean, Simon, and Lucie. Lou was interred at Arlington National Cemetery in Section 60, stone 9936, and was post-humously awarded the Bronze Star with Valor and the Purple Heart.

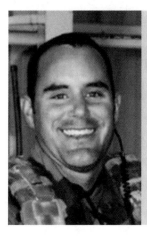

CHIEF PETTY OFFICER MATTHEW MASON

Photo Credit: Sandiegouniontribune.com // US Navy

Matt was raised in Holt, Missouri, just north of Kansas City. He attended Maple Woods Community College and graduated from Northwest Missouri State University in 1998. The following year, Matt enlisted in the Navy and qualified as an information systems technician before entering Basic Underwater Demolition/SEAL training. After finishing the Basic Airborne Course and SEAL Qualification Training in 2001, he reported to SEAL Team ONE and served with the unit for three years. Matt was then assigned to SEAL Team THREE until he received his final orders to the Naval Special Warfare Development Group in June 2006. During his military career, he deployed seven times to support Operations Iraqi Freedom and Enduring Freedom.

On August 6, 2011, Chief Petty Officer Matthew Mason, 37, was killed in Afghanistan when the helicopter he was on board was shot down by enemy fire. He is survived by his widow, Jessica; his three sons; his parents; and his brother, Michael. Matt was laid to rest in Arlington National Cemetery in Section 60, stone 9932; he was posthumously decorated with several commendations, including the Bronze Star with Valor and the Purple Heart.

The Matt Mason Memorial Cowboy Up! Triathlon is held annually in Missouri. The memorial event raises funds for two scholarships awarded in Matt's name, as well as a number of other veterans' organizations. To register for the race or make a contribution, please visit www.CowboyUpTriathlon.com.

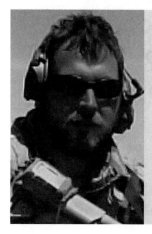

CHIEF PETTY OFFICER STEPHEN MILLS

Photo Credit: Goatlocker.org

Stephen "Matt" Mills was born in Austin, Texas, and graduated from Martin High School in Arlington. He began active duty in the Navy in 1997 and initially served as an operations specialist aboard the USS Kinkaid (DD-965). Three years later, Matt left for Basic Underwater Demolition/SEAL training and finished the course in June 2001. He received orders to SEAL Team THREE in Coronado, California and deployed in 2003 to Iraq. After successfully screening for the Naval Special Warfare Development Group, Matt relocated to the East Coast and worked as a close quarters combat instructor. He was assigned to Tactical Evaluation and Development Squadron THREE in 2006 and went on to complete multiple deployments in support of Operation Enduring Freedom.

Matt married his fiancée in 2011, shortly before returning to Afghanistan. Chief Petty Officer Stephen Mills, 35, was killed in the helicopter crash on August 6. He is survived by his widow, Keri; his children, Cash, Bryce, and Zoe; his parents, Steve and Cheryl; and his siblings, Michael and Ashley.

At Arlington National Cemetery, Matt was interred alongside many of his teammates in Section 60, stone 9933. He had often visited his family in Bastrop, Texas while on leave and, in 2013, the town dedicated a bridge across the Colorado River in his memory. Matt's widow also started the Matt Mills One Fight Fund, which helps the survivors of fallen service members by covering immediate expenses after their loss. To make a donation in Matt's name, please visit www.Charity Smith.org/Endeavors/MMills.

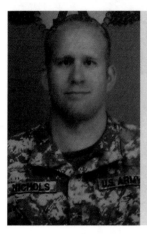

CHIEF WARRANT OFFICER 2 BRYAN NICHOLS

Photo Credit: Veterantributes.com

Bryan was raised in Hays, Kansas, and was the son of a Chinook helicopter pilot who had served during Vietnam. He enlisted in the Army Reserve before graduating high school in 1998, and served as a medical supply specialist with the 388th Medical Logistics Battalion in his hometown. In March 2006, Bryan was appointed a Warrant Officer and assigned to Company B, 7th Battalion, 158th Aviation Regiment. He then began training as a Rotary Wing Aviator and completed Chinook flight qualifications in June 2008. Though he had already served overseas, Bryan was eager to fly and volunteered to mobilize for deployment.

On August 6, 2011, Chief Warrant Officer 2 Bryan Nichols, 31, was serving as the pilot in command of the Chinook when it was shot down in Afghanistan. He is survived by his widow, Mary; his son, Braydon; his parents, Douglas and Cynthia; and his siblings, Monte, Brandon, and Nicole. Bryan was posthumously decorated with the Bronze Star and the Purple Heart for his meritorious service.

While driving through Kansas, the band Little Texas encountered miles of road lined by people holding American flags. They soon found out they had arrived ahead of the funeral procession for Bryan, and the experience inspired their song "Slow Ride Home". A memorial fund was established in Bryan's name through the Endowment Foundation at Thomas More Prep-Marian; donations can be sent to: Bryan J. Nichols Memorial Fund, c/o TMP-Marian Endowment Foundation, 1701 Hall Street, Hays, Kansas 67601.

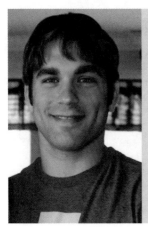

CHIEF PETTY OFFICER NICHOLAS NULL

Photo Credit: Findagrave.com

Nick grew up in West Virginia, and graduated from Parkersburg South High School in 1999. He began taking classes at West Virginia University at Parkersburg but left to enlist in the Navy as a gunner's mate. While assigned to Explosive Ordnance Disposal Mobile Unit SIX in Panama City, Florida, Nick deployed overseas and took part in combat missions during the opening stages of Operation Iraqi Freedom. He then entered the Explosive Ordnance Disposal training program and graduated in 2004 and was stationed with EOD Mobile Unit TWO in Virginia Beach. Nick spent four years working with the unit before receiving order to the Naval Special Warfare Development Group in January 2009. He completed multiple deployments to the Middle East during his military service and earned the designation of master EOD technician.

On August 6, 2011 Chief (Select) Nicholas Null, 30, was killed when the helicopter he was on board was shot down by enemy fire. He is survived by his widow, Tanya; their sons, Hunter, Brett, and Chase; his mother, Tracy Litman; his father, Timothy Null; and his siblings, Ashley Sanders and Brandon Null. Nick, having already selected for Chief, was promoted to the rank posthumously.

The Nick Null Memorial Foundation was established by Nick's mother to honor his memory and support other veteran service organizations. Donations can be sent to: The Nick Null Memorial Foundation, 1049 Lake Washington Road, Washington, WV 26181.

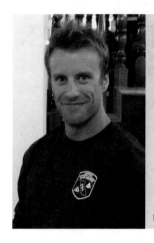

PETTY OFFICER FIRST CLASS JESSE PITTMAN

Photo Credit: Pritzkermilitary.com

Jesse grew up in Willits, a small town in northern California. He graduated from high school in 2002 and spent three years working as a seasonal fire fighter before enlisting in the Navy. After completing Basic Underwater Demolition/SEAL training and the Basic Airborne Course in 2007, Jesse reported to SEAL Team FIVE. He gained a reputation for his bull-headed sense of determination and attacking every challenge that came at him. Jesse was often heard saying, "I don't run, I charge." At one point he contemplated leaving combat to earn his degree and become an officer but instead volunteered for an additional deployment. Jesse had already deployed multiple times to the Middle East to support Operation Enduring Freedom and, in 2011, left for Afghanistan as an individual augmentee to the Navy Special Warfare Development Group.

On August 6, Petty Officer First Class Jesse Pittman, 27, was on board the helicopter when it was struck by a rocket-propelled grenade. He is survived by his parents, J. Terry and Ida; and his brothers, J. Terry Jr. and Corey. He was posthumously decorated with the Bronze Star with Valor and the Purple Heart.

The Jesse Pittman Memorial Fund provides tuition to Mendocino County students cut from the same cloth as Jesse: that of determination and hard work. The scholarships are funded by donations and an annual 5k run/walk. Direct contributions can be made at www.CommunityFound.org; for additional information on the scholarship and event, please visit www.JessePittmanFund.org.

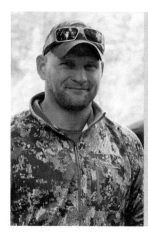

SENIOR CHIEF PETTY OFFICER THOMAS RATZLAFF

Photo Credit: Arkansasrunforthefallen.org

Tommy was raised in Green Forest, Arkansas and enlisted in the Navy in 1995. Initially trained as a gunner's mate, he served two years aboard the USS Kidd (DDG-993) before entering Basic Underwater Demolition/SEAL training. Tommy reported to SEAL Team TWO in 1999, and spent four years with the unit before successfully screening for the Naval Special Warfare Development Group.

During his military service, Tommy completed multiple deployments overseas to Kosovo and the Middle East. On November 28, 2008, he was in Afghanistan working alongside Canadian military when their assault force encountered a machine gun nest. Tommy faced almost point blank fire to neutralize the enemy, and was credited with saving multiple lives. He was later awarded the Canadian Star of Military Valor, which has been given to only one other American since WWI.

Senior Chief Petty Officer Thomas Ratzlaff, 34, was on board the Chinook when it was downed by enemy fire on August 6, 2011. He is survived by his widow, their three children, his mother, and his sister; his father passed away in 2010. Tommy was laid to rest in Arlington National Cemetery in Section 60, at stone 9935, and received the Bronze Star with Valor and the Purple Heart.

The Ratzlaff Legacy Foundation was created to honor Tommy and supports several local organizations. The foundation hosts an annual memorial walk/run and maintains the Tommy Ratzlaff Scholarship Fund. To sign up for the 5k or make a contribution, please visit www.RatzLegacy.org.

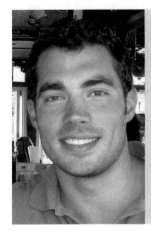

CHIEF PETTY OFFICER ROBERT REEVES

Photo Credit: Arlingtoncemetery.net

Rob was raised in Shreveport, Louisiana and attended Caddo Magnet School. He played lacrosse and shared the soccer field with his teammate, Jonas Kelsall, who he later served alongside in the military. Rob graduated in 1997 and spent a year at Louisiana State University before enlisting in the Navy. After finishing Basic Underwater Demolition/SEAL training and the Basic Airborne Course, he received orders to SEAL Team FIVE and, later served with SEAL Team SEVEN. Rob selected for the Naval Special Warfare Development Group in 2004. During his military service, he completed multiple deployments to Iraq and Afghanistan to support the Global War on Terror.

Chief Petty Officer Robert Reeves, 32, was killed in Afghanistan when his helicopter was struck by a rocket-propelled grenade on August 6, 2011. He is survived by his father, Jim; and his sister, Emily; his mother, Sherry, passed away in 2007. In accordance with his wishes, Rob was buried at sea; a cenotaph bearing his name can be found in Arlington National Cemetery, in Section MK, stone 265. He was posthumously awarded several honors, including the Bronze Star with Valor and the Purple Heart.

Rob's family requested memorial donations be made to either the Wounded Warrior Project or the Navy SEAL Foundation; both organizations provide support to military personnel and their families. To learn more about their programs or to make a contribution, please visit www.WoundedWarrior Project.org and www.Navy SEALFoundation.org.

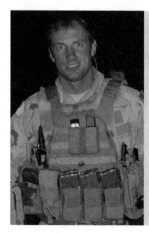

CHIEF PETTY OFFICER AARON VAUGHN

Photo Credit: Sandiegouniontribune.com // US Navy

Aaron was born in Obion County, Tennessee and was raised on a small farm near Union City. At only eight years old, he declared his plans to become a Navy SEAL. Aaron enlisted in the Navy on his twenty-first birthday and, graduated from Basic Underwater Demolition/SEAL training in April 2004. After completing his advance qualifications, he was assigned to SEAL Team ONE in Coronado, California. Aaron later worked as an instructor at the Naval Special Warfare Group ONE Training Detachment and, in October 2010, reported to the Naval Special Warfare Development Group in Virginia Beach. Over the course of his career, Aaron would serve overseas in Germany and Guam and completed multiple deployments to the Middle East.

Petty Officer First Class Aaron Vaughn, 30, was killed in the Chinook crash on August 6, 2011. He is survived by his widow, Kimberley; their children, Reagan and Chamberlyn; his parents, Billy and Karen; and his sisters, Tara and Ana. Aaron was interred with many of his teammates at Arlington National Cemetery in Section 60, stone 9927. For his honorable service, he was posthumously promoted to the rank of Chief Petty Officer and received several medals, including the Bronze Star with Valor and the Purple Heart.

Operation 300 was founded to honor Aaron's memory and the families of the fallen. The organization is dedicated to children who have lost their fathers as a result of military service. To make a contribution or to sign up for an event, please visit them at www.Operation300.com.

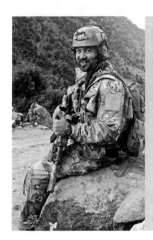

SENIOR CHIEF PETTY OFFICER KRAIG VICKERS

Photo Credit: Sandiegouniontribune.com // US Navy

Kraig was born and raised in Hawaii. After graduating from Maui High School in 1992, he began attending Evangel College in Missouri on a football scholarship. Kraig soon decided college wasn't where he was supposed to be and returned home to work a few odd jobs. He decided to enlist in the Navy in 21996 and qualified as an Explosive Ordnance Disposal technician two years later. Kraig was first assigned to EOD Mobile Unit FIVE in Guam, and later served with EOD Mobile Unit EIGHT in Bahrain and Mobile Unit THREE in Hawaii before. He then reported to the Naval Special Warfare Development Group in 2005 and went on to complete multiple deployments to Iraq and Afghanistan. At home, Kraig was a dedicated family man who loved spending time with his children and maintained a strong faith in God.

On August 6, 2011, Senior Chief Petty Officer Kraig Vickers, 36, was on board the Chinook helicopter when it was shot down by a rocket-propelled grenade. He is survived by his widow, Nani; his children, Makahea, Kala'i, Malie, and Kalei; his parents, Robert Sr. and Mary; his brothers, Robert Jr., Mark, and Vance; and his sister, Michelle.

Just a few days after his death, over 200 surfers and stand-up paddlers gathered off the shore of Virginia Beach to remember Kraig with a paddle-out ceremony. In Maui, the Kraig Vickers Honor Run is held annually to keep his memory alive. Please visit the "Kraig Vickers Honor Run" Facebook page for more information on registering for the event.

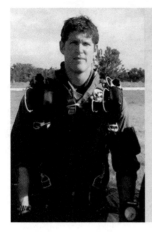

CHIEF PETTY OFFICER JASON WORKMAN

Photo Credit: Goatlocker.org

Jason was brought up in Blanding, Utah and graduated from San Juan High School in 1997. He spent the next two years in Philadelphia and Belo Horizonte, Brazil as a full-time missionary for the Church of Jesus Christ of Latter-day Saints. After earning his criminal justice degree from Southern Utah University in 2003, Jason enlisted in the Navy with the intent to become a SEAL. He entered Basic Underwater Demolition/SEAL training in January 2004, and finished his advance training the following year. Jason was assigned to SEAL Team TWO in Virginia Beach for three years before receiving orders to the Naval Special Warfare Development Group. He completed multiple deployments to the Middle East during his career, and returned overseas to serve in Afghanistan in 2011.

On August 6 of that year, Petty Officer First Class Jason Workman, 32, was killed in the Chinook crash. He is survived by his widow, Stacey; their son, Jax; his parents, Rodney and Betty; and his brothers, Corey, Stephen, and Timothy. Jason was interred at Arlington National Cemetery in Section 60, stone 9928, and was posthumously promoted to the rank of Chief Petty Officer.

At his funeral, Jason's family requested donations in his name be made to the Navy SEAL Foundation. Dedicated to those serving in Naval Special Warfare and their families, the foundation has provided assistance and support to the community since 2000. Please visit www.NavySEALFoundation.org to make a contribution.

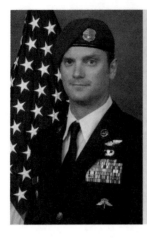

TECHNICAL SERGEANT DANIEL ZERBE

Photo Credit: Veterantributes.org

Daniel grew up in the small Pennsylvania town of Red Lion. He enlisted after graduating high school in 2001, and began pursuing his place in Special Forces. Daniel qualified as a Pararescueman and, in 2003, was assigned to the 38th Rescue Squadron at Moody Air Force Base, Georgia. Three years later, he received orders to the 24th Special Tactics Squadron at Pope Air Force Base, North Carolina, where he remained for the rest of his career. Daniel loved his job and, across multiple deployments to Afghanistan and Iraq, proved his dedication to the PJs' credo, "That others may live." In 2010, Daniel was recognized as the Air Force Pararescueman Non-Commissioned Officer of the Year.

Technical Sergeant Daniel Zerbe, 28, was killed on August 6, 2011 when the helicopter he was on board was shot down in Afghanistan. He is survived by his parents, Terry and Sue Zerbe; his siblings, Christopher and Megan; and his girlfriend, Amanda Harke. Daniel was interred at Arlington National Cemetery in Section 60, stone 9940, alongside many of the men with whom he fought and died.

In Daniel's hometown, an annual ride is held to raise money for a memorial scholarship in his name; for more information please visit the "Tech. Sgt. Daniel Lee Zerbe Memorial Event" Facebook page. Please also consider making a contribution to the That Others May Live Foundation; since 2002 they have been dedicated to providing emergency financial assistance and tuition funds to the families of fallen and injured Air Force Rescue Airmen. Read more at www.ThatOthersMayLive.org.

CHIEF PETTY OFFICER BRIAN BILL

Brian was a SEAL assigned to the Naval Special Warfare Development Group, and has been memorialized with his own workout; his story can be found on page 178.

PETTY OFFICER FIRST CLASS JOHN DOUANGDARA & MILITARY WORKING DOG BART

John and his canine, Bart, were assigned to the Naval Special Warfare Development Group to support combat operations. To learn more about the canine handling team, please see the workout dedicated to them on page 180.

CHIEF PETTY OFFICER JOHN FAAS

John was a SEAL assigned to the Naval Special Warfare Development Group; to see the workout dedicated to him and to read his story, please go to page 182.

STAFF SERGEANT ANDREW HARVELL

Andy was a Combat Controller serving with the 24th Special Tactics Squadron. To read more about him and the workout dedicated to his memory, please see page 184.

LIEUTENANT COMMANDER JONAS KELSALL

Jonas served as a SEAL troop commander and was assigned to the Naval Special Warfare Development Group. The workout dedicated to him can be found with his biography on page 186.

CHIEF PETTY OFFICER HEATH ROBINSON

Heath was a SEAL assigned to the Naval Special Warfare Development Group; the workout named after him can be found with his biography on page 188.

PETTY OFFICER SECOND CLASS NICHOLAS SPEHAR

Nick was a SEAL assigned to SEAL Team FIVE during Operation Red Wings, and was honored with an individual workout. His section starts on page 190.

PETTY OFFICER FIRST CLASS MICHAEL STRANGE

Mike was a Cryptologic Technician assigned to Naval Special Warfare Development Group to support combat operations. He has been honored with a workout in his name, which can be found on page 192.

CHIEF PETTY OFFICER JON TUMILSON

Jon was a SEAL assigned to the Naval Special Warfare Development Group, and has been memorialized with an individual workout; his story is on page 194.

"People sleep peaceably in their beds at night only because rough men stand ready to do violence on their behalf."

George Orwell

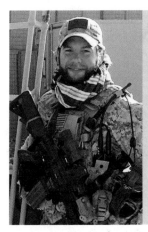

CHIEF PETTY OFFICER BRIAN BILL
August 6, 2011

Photo Credit: Crossfit

Born and raised in Stamford, Connecticut. Following his graduation from Trinity Catholic High School in 1997, he joined the Corps of Cadets at Norwich University and earned his degree in electrical engineering. Brian enlisted in the Navy in 2001 and entered Basic Underwater Demolition/ SEAL training that November. In June 2003, he reported to SEAL Team EIGHT and served with the unit for years. Brian was then selected to serve with the Naval Special Warfare Development Group and relocated to Virginia Beach.

During his military service, Brian completed multiple combat deployments to the Middle East. He was deployed to Afghanistan in 2010 when his teammate, Chief Petty Officer Adam Brown, was mortally wounded in a firefight (page 152). Brian risked his life that day to try and save Adam, and his extraordinary heroism later recognized with the Bronze Star with Valor.

Chief Petty Officer (Select) Brian Bill, 31, was killed on August 6, 2011 when the helicopter he was on board was shot down in Afghanistan. He is survived by his mother and stepfather, Patricia and Michael Parry; his father, Scott Bill; and his siblings, Christian, Morgan, Amy, Andrea, Kerry, and Tessa. Brian was interred at Arlington National Cemetery in Section 60, stone 9930; having been selected for Chief prior to his death, Brian was promoted to the rank posthumously. Please see page 152 to read more about Extortion 17.

To honor her brother's legacy, Brian's sister Amy started The Little Warriors, an organization dedicated to the children of fallen Navy SEALs; visit their website at www.NavySEALLittleWarriors.org.

BRIAN

3 rounds for time:
5 ROPE CLIMBS (15')
25 BACK SQUATS (185lbs)

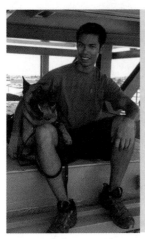

PETTY OFFICER FIRST CLASS JOHN DOUANGDARA & MILITARY WORKING DOG BART

August 6, 2011

Photo Credit: Veterantributes.org

John was raised in South Sioux City, Nebraska and enlisted in the Navy as a master-at-arms. John attended the canine handling course John attended the canine handling course and, in 2005, completed his first deployment to the Middle East. He then spent two years assigned to Naval Submarine Base New London in Connecticut before receiving orders to the Naval Special Warfare Development Group. John became a Combat Assault Dog Handler in 2008, and deployed multiple times to Afghanistan to support SEAL team operations. One of his dogs, Toby, saved the lives of six Canadian service members at the cost of his own; both John and Toby were later recognized by the Canadian military for their heroic actions.

On August 6, 2011, Petty Officer First Class John Douangdara, 26, and his Military Working Dog, Bart, were killed when the Chinook they were on board was shot down by enemy fire in Afghanistan. John is survived by his parents, Phouthasith and Sengchanh; and four brothers and sisters. At Arlington National Cemetery, he was laid to rest with many of his teammates in Section 60, stone 9926. John was posthumously awarded the Bronze Star with Valor and the Purple Heart. Please see page 152 to read the story of Extortion 17.

To make a contribution in memory of John and Bart, please consider the Military Working Dog Team Support Association, a charitable organization dedicated to handlers and their dogs; visit their website at www.MWDTSA.org.

DOUANGDARA + BART

5 rounds with a partner, for time:

BEAR CRAWL (50M)

Each partner completes the following, alternating after each rep:

8 BURPEE BOX JUMPS (30"/24")

6 SQUAT CLEANS (155/105lbs)

11 WALL BALL SHOTS (20/10lbs)

4 SLED PUSH (50M 45/25lbs)

[source unknown]

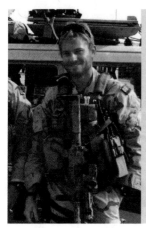

CHIEF PETTY OFFICER JOHN FAAS
August 6, 2011

Photo Credit: Goatlocker.org

John was raised in Minneapolis, and graduated from Minnehaha Academy in 1998. Despite having many options for college, he spent a year preparing for the physical trials faced by Navy SEALs and enlisted in the Navy; John successfully finished Basic Underwater Demolition/SEAL training and his advanced qualifications in 2001. He was initially stationed with SEAL Team EIGHT in Virginia Beach, and served overseas in Germany, the Horn of Africa, and Afghanistan while assigned to the unit. In 2005, John was selected for a position with the Naval Special Warfare Development Group and went on to complete multiple deployments to the Middle East.

Throughout his life, John pushed himself to be excellent. In addition to intense physical training, he meditated and challenged his mind with classical literature, religious texts, and books on warfare. John also devoted much of his spare time to the pursuit of a bachelor's degree.

On August 6, 2011, Chief Petty Officer John Faas, 31, was killed when the helicopter he was on board was shot down by a rocket-propelled grenade. He is survived by his parents, Robert and Gretchen Faas, and was posthumously decorated with the Bronze Star with Valor and the Purple Heart. To read the story of Extortion 17, please see page 152.

The John Faas Foundation was created to honor his memory; the organization maintains an education endowment fund, and grants scholarships to Naval Special Warfare service members and their families. Go to www.JohnFaasFountation.com to make a contribution.

FAAS FIT

3 rounds for time:

10 DEADLIFTS (315/215lbs)

20 PULL-UPS

30 KB SNATCHES (1.5/1 pood)

Courtesy of The 31Heroes Project

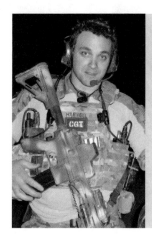

STAFF SERGEANT ANDREW HARVELL

August 6, 2011

Photo Credit: Harvellfund.com

Andy grew up in Long Beach, California and attended Miliken High School. He enlisted in the Air Force after his graduation in 1992, and entered the training pipeline to become a Combat Controller. Andy spent two years qualifying as a CCT, and another completing the advanced tactical courses required for Special Operations. In 2006, he reported to the 21st Special Tactics Squadron at Pope Field, North Carolina and completed four deployments to the Middle East over the next three years. Andy was then assigned to the 24th Special Tactics Squadron and, in 2011, began his second deployment with the unit in support of Operation Enduring Freedom.

Staff Sergeant Andrew Harvell, 26, was killed when the Chinook he was on board was shot down by a rocket-propelled grenade on August 6, 2011. He leaves behind his widow, Krista; their sons, Hunter and Ethan; his parents, John and Jane; and his siblings, Sean and Analese. Staff Sergeant Sean Harvell escorted his brother's body home, where over 100 Combat Controllers and Pararescuemen attended Andy's funeral to pay their respects. The story of Extortion 17 can be found on page 152.

In his memory, Andy's friends built the "Big Andy" workout and now host an annual event to raise funds for Hunter and Ethan's educational trust. The organizers also encourage donations be made to the Special Operations Warrior Foundation to help secure college education for the children of other fallen service members; to learn more, please visit www.HarvellFund.com.

BIG ANDY

With a partner and only one person working at a time, complete 2 rounds for time:

11 ROPE CLIMBS
(OR 50 PULL-UPS)

BUDDY CARRY (200M)

33 POWER CLEANS (135/95lbs)

BUDDY CARRY (400M)

55 FRONT SQUATS (135/95lbs)

66 BURPEES*

Workout Notes
*With double push-up

Courtesy of the Harvell Fund

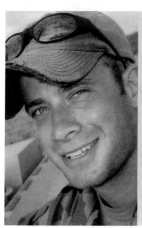

LIEUTENANT COMMANDER JONAS KELSALL

August 6, 2011

Photo Credit: Arlingtoncemetery.net

Jonas was born and raised in Shreveport, Louisiana. He enlisted in the Navy after his graduation from Caddo Magnet School in 1996 and finished Basic Underwater Demolition/SEAL training the following year. Jonas was then able to attend the University of Texas to earn his degree as a ROTC cadet. After receiving his commission in 2001, he reported to SEAL Team SEVEN in Coronado; Jonas remained with the command until 2008, when he was assigned to the Naval Special Warfare Development Group as a troop commander. He completed multiple deployment to the Middle East during his military service and, in 2011, returned to Afghanistan to support Operation Enduring Freedom.

On August 6, Lieutenant Jonas Kelsall, 32, was killed when the helicopter he was on board was shot down by enemy. He is survived by his widow, Victoria; his parents, John and Teri; and his sister, Kim. Jonas was laid to rest with many of his teammates at Arlington National Cemetery in Section 60, stone 9937, and was posthumously decorated with the Bronze Star with Valor and the Purple Heart.

After his death, Victoria established the Jonas B. Kelsall Memorial Fund, which has provided assistance to the families affected by the crash of Extortion 17; donations can be made at www.JonasBKelsall MemorialFund.org. Additionally, Jonas' parents started the Jonas Project to fulfill the dreams their son had of giving back—the organization works to create jobs by providing support and growing veteran-owned businesses. To learn more, please visit www.TheJonasProject.org.

THE JONAS PROJECT MEMORIAL WOD

For time:

ROW (1000M)

Then, 3 rounds:

11 BENCH PRESSES*

8 SUICIDES (10M)

3 ROPE CLIMBS

32 TOE-TOUCHES**

ROW (1000M)

Workout Notes
*Lbs equal to body weight
**On a slam ball

Courtesy of The 31 Heroes Project

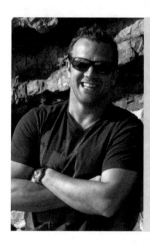

SENIOR CHIEF PETTY OFFICER HEATH ROBINSON

August 6, 2011

Photo Credit: Arlingtoncemetery.net

Heath was raised in the northern Michigan town of Petoskey and graduated high school in 1995. The following year, he enlisted in the Navy
and entered Basic Underwater Demolition/SEAL training. Heath did not
finish the course and reported to Amphibious Group ONE in Okinawa,
Japan. After two years spent working as an operations specialist, Heath
was granted a second chance at BUD/S and successfully completed the
training. He went on to serve with SEAL Teams THREE and SEVEN and,
in 2004, was selected for an assignment with the Naval Special Warfare
Development Group. Heath deployed to the Middle East multiple times
during his military service, and returned to Afghanistan with his team
in 2011.

On August 6, 2011, Senior Chief Petty Officer Heath Robinson, 34,
was killed in the line of duty when the Chinook he was on board was hit
by rocket-propelled grenade. He is survived by his widow and two daughters; his mother, Deborah Robinson-Coxe; his father, Dan Robinson; and
his two brothers. Heath was laid to rest with many of his teammates in
Arlington National Cemetery, and can be found in Section 60, stone 9934.
Read more about the story of Extortion 17 on page 152.

In memory of Heath, a bridge in the Upper Peninsula of Michigan was
rededicated as the Heath Michael Robinson Cut River Memorial Bridge.
A scholarship was also established in his name by the Petoskey-Harbor
Springs Area Community Foundation. To make a donation, please visit
www.PHSACF.org/Donate-106/.

HEATH

7 rounds for time:

7 SUMO DEADLIFT HIGH-PULLS (95/65lbs)

7 POWER SNATCHES (95/65lbs)

7 OVERHEAD SQUATS (95/65lbs)

[source unknown].

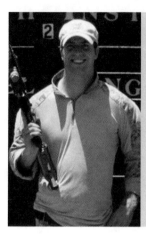

PETTY OFFICER SECOND CLASS NICHOLAS SPEHAR

August 6, 2011

Photo Credit: Sandiegouniontribune.com // US Navy

Nick grew up in Chisago City, Minnesota, where he attended Chisago Lakes High School. Nick was a gifted student-athlete: he lettered academically and was a member of the school's football, baseball, and swim teams. After graduating in 2005, he began working in construction and welding but knew he ultimately wanted to become a SEAL. He enlisted in the Navy in 2007, then entered the rigorous qualification program required of SEALs. Nick completed Basic Underwater Demolition/SEAL training and advanced qualifications the following year and was assigned to SEAL Team FIVE in Coronado, California.

Over the next few years, Nick would serve tours of duty in the Philippines and Yemen in support of Operation Enduring Freedom. He then volunteered to augment the Naval Special Warfare Development Group for a deployment to Afghanistan in 2011. Petty Officer Second Class Nicholas Spehar, 24, lost his life when the helicopter he was on was brought down by enemy fire on August 6. He is survived by his parents, Patrick and Anette; and his siblings, Marie, Lisa, Luke, and Jacob. To read more about the story of Extortion 17, please see page 152.

Near Nick's hometown in Minnesota, a stretch of U.S. Highway 8 was designated the Nicholas Patrick Spehar Memorial Highway in his honor. Additionally, the Nicholas Spehar Memorial Scholarship is a full-ride scholarship awarded to students at Holy Cross College in Notre Dame, Indiana. To make a donation in Nick's name, please visit www.College Relations.HCC-ND.edu/Give.

SPEHAR

For time:

100 THRUSTERS (135lbs)

100 CHEST-TO-BAR PULL-UPS

RUN (6 MILES)

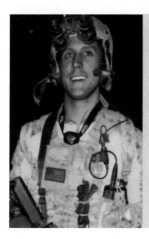

PETTY OFFICER FIRST CLASS MICHAEL STRANGE

August 6, 2011

Photo Credit: Crossfit

Michael grew up in the Wissinoming neighborhood of Philadelphia, and enlisted in the Navy after his high school graduation in 2004. After completing training as cryptologic technician, he was first stationed at the Navy Information Operations Command in Kunia, Hawaii. Michael later volunteered to augment SEAL Team TWO, and spent nine months supporting combat operations in Iraq. In 2009, he was selected to serve with the Naval Special Warfare Development Group and relocated to Virginia Beach with his girlfriend and their dog, Schmayze.

Petty Officer First Class Michael Strange, 25, was killed on August 6, 2011 when the helicopter he was on board was shot down by enemy fire in Afghanistan. He is survived by his fiancée, Breanna Hostetler; his parents, Charles Jr. and Elizabeth; his brother, Charles III; and his sisters, Katelyn and Carly. Michael was laid to rest at Arlington National Cemetery in Section 60, stone 9925, alongside many of his teammates. In recognition of their service, both Michael and Petty Officer First Class Jared Day were posthumously decorated with the National Intelligence Medal for Valor. The story of Extortion 17 can be found on page 152.

After his death, Michael's family started the Michael Strange Foundation to provide unconditional support to fallen service members and their families. One of their major initiatives is hosting retreats to create a healing environment for Gold Star families. Please visit www.MichaelStrangeFoundation.org to make a contribution in honor of Michael's sacrifice.

STRANGE

8 rounds for time:

RUN (600M)

11 WEIGHTED PULL-UPS*

11 WALKING LUNGE STEPS*

11 KB THRUSTERS*

Workout Notes
*With 1.5 pood kettlebells

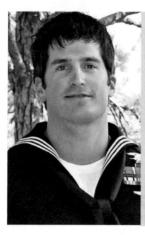

CHIEF PETTY OFFICER JON TUMILSON
August 6, 2011

Photo Credit: Sandiegouniontribune.com // US Navy

Jon "JT" Tumilson grew up in the small town of Rockford, Iowa. He committed himself to becoming a Navy SEAL at the age of 15, and left for boot camp shortly after graduating high school in 1995. After five years spent serving as an operation specialist aboard the USS Port Royal (CG-73), JT was selected to begin training as a SEAL. He went on to serve with three West Coast units before receiving orders to the Naval Special Warfare Development Group in August 2009, and completed multiple deployments to the Middle East throughout his military career.

Petty Officer First Class Jon Tumilson, 35, was killed when the helicopter he was on board was shot down by a rocket-propelled grenade on August 6, 2011. He leaves behind his father, George; his sisters, Kristie and Joy; and his beloved dog, Hawkeye; his mother, Cathy, passed away in 2015. For his dedicated service, JT was posthumously promoted to the rank of Chief Petty Officer, and was awarded the Bronze Star with Valor and the Purple Heart. To read more about Extortion 17, please see page 152.

JT's hometown hosts the annual Jon Tumilson Go Crush It 5k Challenge, where hundreds of residents turn out to remember a local hero. More information on the run and other events can be found on the "In Memory of Navy SEAL Jon Tumilson" Facebook page. Donations in JT's name may also be made to the Navy SEAL Foundation; visit them at www.NavySEALFoundation.org.

TUMILSON

8 rounds for time:

RUN (200M)

11 DUMBBELL BURPEE DEADLIFTS*

Workout Notes
*With 60lbs dumbbells

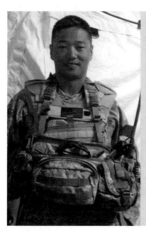

MAJOR WALTER DAVID GRAY
August 8, 2012

Photo Credit: Crossfit // fingagrave.com

Walter David Gray was raised in Conyers, Georgia; he graduated from Loganville High School in 1992, and later enlisted in the Air Force. Initially trained as a Tactical Air Control Party member, David joined the ROTC program at Charleston Southern College and earned his bachelor's degree in 2001. He continued his career in the Air Force as an officer, and initially worked as an airfield operations officer. The opportunity arose for David to return to the TACP training program and he graduated in the first class to integrate officers.

David was assigned to the 13th Air Support Operations Squadron, 93rd Air Ground Operations Wing in Fort Carson, Colorado when he deployed to Afghanistan in 2012. On August 8, Major David Gray was killed by the detonation of a second bomb; the attack took the lives of two other service members. He is survived by his widow, Heather; and by their children, Nyah, Garrett, and Ava. David was posthumously decorated with the Bronze Star with Valor, and interred at Arlington National Cemetery in Section 60, stone 9091-A.

Thirteen of the men who served with David in Afghanistan honored him with a memorial ruck march in 2013. Starting at Dover Air Force Base in Delaware, they traced the 140-mile route his body traveled to Arlington National Cemetery. Please consider making a donation in his name to the TACP Association; the organization is dedicated to supporting TACP members and their families in times of need. Visit their website at www.USATACP.org.

DG

In 10 minutes, as many rounds as possible:

8 TOES-TO-BAR

8 DUMBBELL THRUSTERS*

12 WALKING LUNGE STEPS*

Workout Notes

*With 35lbs dumbbells

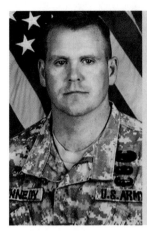

MAJOR
THOMAS KENNEDY

August 8, 2012

Photo Credit: Crossfit

Tom grew up in New City, New York and attended Don Bosco Preparatory School. As a cadet at the United States Military Academy at West Point, he played hockey for the Black Knights and commissioned in the Army in 2000. He deployed twice to Iraq before his selection for instructor duty at West Point; as a tactical officer, Tom was responsible for educating and mentoring future Army officers. He received his next assignment to Headquarters and Headquarters Company, 4th Brigade Combat Team, 4th Infantry Division and reported to Fort Carson, Colorado.

On August 8, 2012, Major Thomas Kennedy, 35, was serving overseas in Afghanistan when he was killed by a suicide bomber; the Taliban claimed responsibility for the attack, which also took the lives of two other service members. Tom leaves behind his widow, Kami; their children, Brody and Margaret; his parents, George and Patricia; and his brothers, John and George. He was posthumously awarded the Bronze Star and the Purple Heart, and laid to rest at the Post Cemetery at West Point.

Don Bosco Preparatory High School established a scholarship in Tom's name. They also host an annual memorial hockey game and give the TK Award to the player who best exemplifies his leadership and values; Tom's jersey, no. 10, was retired at the inaugural game in 2013. For more information, go to www.DonBosco Hockey.com/TK/. Contributions in memory of Tom can be made to the school at www.DonBoscoPrep.org/Pages/Offices-Pages/Advancement/Donate-Online.

TK

In 20 minutes, as many rounds as possible:

8 PULL-UPS*

8 BOX JUMPS (36")

12 KB SWINGS (2 pood)

Workout Notes
*Strict pull-ups

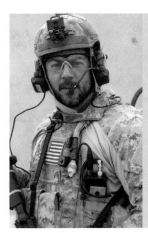

CHIEF PETTY OFFICER COLLIN THOMAS
August 18, 2010

Photo Credit: Findagrave.com

Collin was a native of Morehead, Kentucky, and became a cadet in the Army ROTC program at Morehead State University. In 1997, he left college to enlist in the Navy. Collin qualified as a hospital corpsman before entering Basic Underwater Demolition/SEAL Training in 1998. He went on to spend six years working with SEAL Teams FOUR and TWO in Virginia Beach and, in 2006, was selected to serve with the Naval Special Warfare Development Group. During his military service, Collin completed at least eight deployments to trans-Sahara Africa and the Middle East.

Collin's family was rarely given the details of his location or his work, but knew that in 2010 he was deployed to eastern Afghanistan. On August 18, Colling was leading an assault against a Taliban cell when he realized the enemy's entrenched position was a danger to his team. Chief Petty Officer Collin Thomas, 33, moved to flank the insurgents and was fatally shot while eliminating the threat. He is survived by his fiancée, Sarah Saunders; his parents, Clay and Paula; his sister, Meghan; and his dog, Hagan. In recognition of his courageous actions, Collin was posthumously decorated with the Silver Star and was laid to rest in his hometown with full military honors.

Collin's family requested memorial donations be made to the Navy SEAL Foundation, an organization dedicated to Naval Special Warfare service members and their families. To make a contribution, please visit www.NavySEALFoundation.org.

COLLIN

6 rounds for time:

SANDBAG CARRY (400M 50lbs)

12 PUSH PRESSES (115lbs)

12 BOX JUMPS (24")

12 SUMO DEADLIFT HIGH-PULLS (95lbs)

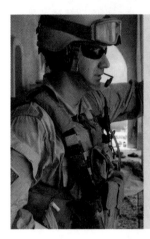

SERGEANT FIRST CLASS MICHAEL TULLY

August 23, 2007

Photo Credit: Crossfit

After growing up in Falls Creek, Pennsylvania, Michael enlisted in the Marine Corps in 1993 and qualified as a reconnaissance diver. He transferred to the Army four years later and was served as an infantryman in Fort Bragg, North Carolina. Michael entered the Special Forces Qualification Course in 2004, where he received training as a combat medic and earned his Green Beret. He was then assigned to Company C, 2nd Battalion, 1st Special Forces Group (Airborne) at Fort Lewis, Washington and began his second deployment to Iraq in 2007.

On August 23, Sergeant First Class Michael Tully, 33, was near Al Aziziyah when the blast of an improvised explosive device struck his vehicle; the detonation took his life and that of another Soldier. Michael is survived by his widow, Heather; his son, Slade; his mother and stepfather, Dolores and Art Newman; his father and stepmother, Jack and Marilyn Tully; and his siblings, John and Heather. Sergeant First Class John Tully was concurrently serving in Iraq and accompanied his brother's body home. In recognition of his service, Michael was posthumously awarded the Bronze Star and the Purple Heart, and was laid to rest in Falls Creek with full military honors.

In 2010, a group of Soldiers and veterans from Joint Base Lewis-McChord took part in a half Ironman triathlon to honor Michael and three other Green Berets. Their team raised more than $20,000 in donations for the Special Operations Warrior Foundation; additionally, Michael's son was a recipient of SOWF scholarship funds.

TULLY

4 rounds for time:

SWIM (200M)

23 DUMBBELL SQUAT CLEANS*

Workout Notes
*With 40lbs dumbbells

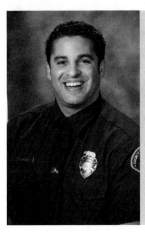

FIREFIGHTER SPECIALIST ARNALDO QUINONES
August 30, 2009

Photo Credit: Findagrave.com

Arnaldo "Arnie" Quinones was born in New York City and moved to California with his family when he was twelve years old. He joined the Los Angeles County Fire Department as a call firefighter in 1998 and graduated from the county fire academy in 2000. Four years later, Arnie was promoted to the rank of Firefighter Specialist and began working with the crew at Camp 16 as Foreman, where he trained and supervised inmate firefighters.

In 2009, a series of wild fires burned across the state of California; the worst of these was the Station Fire north of Los Angeles. The fires reached Camp 16 on August 30, and Firefighter Specialist Arnaldo Quinones and Fire Captain Ted Hall ordered everyone to shelter while they looked for an escape route; the two firefighters were killed when their emergency response vehicle fell 800 feet into a ravine. Their deaths were ruled homicides, as the fires were attributed to arson. Arnie is survived by his widow, Lori; his mother, Sonia; and his brother, Ozzie Jr.; his daughter, Sophia Grace, was born three weeks after her father's death.

The memorial for Arnie and Ted was held at Dodger Stadium; over 15,000 fellow firefighters were in attendance, as well as some of the inmates they had worked to protect. To make a donation in Arnie's name, please consider the National Fallen Firefighters Foundation. Since 1992 they have been committed to honoring firefighters killed in the line of duty and providing support to their families. For more information, please visit www.FireHero.org.

<u>ARNIE</u>

For time, with a single pood kettlebell:

21 TURKISH GET-UPS (RIGHT ARM)

50 KB SWINGS

21 OVERHEAD SQUATS (LEFT ARM)

50 KB SWINGS

21 OVERHEAD SQUATS (RIGHT ARM)

50 KB SWINGS

21 TURKISH GET-UPS (LEFT ARM)

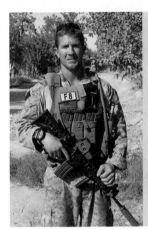

CAPTAIN
JOSHUA MEADOWS
September 5, 2009

Photo Credit: Crossfit

Josh grew up in Elgin, Texas. The son of a Marine, he chose to enlist in the Marine Corps before graduating high school and served as a reservist while earning his business degree at Texas Tech University. Josh commissioned as an officer in 2001 and spent the next two years qualifying as a UH-1N Huey Pilot. During his time in the Marines, Josh completed several tours of duty overseas and was wounded while serving in Iraq. He also deployed aboard the USS Peleliu (LHD-5) in 2008, and saw action as the lead Marine Corps Huey pilot during an operation in the Gulf of Aden. When his military service was done, Josh and his wife had plans to return to Texas and help with the family ranching business.

In November 2008, Josh was recruited for a non-flight special operations assignment; he was stationed with 1st Marine Special Operations Battalion at Camp Pendleton, California and deployed to Afghanistan the following year. On September 5, 2009, Captain Joshua Meadows, 30, was killed by enemy fire during combat operations. He is survived by his widow, Angela; his mother, Jan; and his sister, Erin; his daughter, Olivia, was born after his death. For his courageous service, Josh was posthumously decorated with the Bronze Star with Valor and a second Purple Heart.

To make a donation in Josh's name, please consider the MARSOC Foundation. Dedicated to MARSOC personnel and their families, their organization has provided over $1 million in assistance to date. Visit them at www.MARSOCFoundation.org.

MEADOWS

For time:

20 MUSCLE-UPS

25 LOWERS FROM AN INVERTED HANG ON RINGS*

30 RING HANDSTAND PUSH-UPS

35 RING ROWS

40 RING PUSH-UPS

Workout Notes
*Slowly, with a straight body and arms

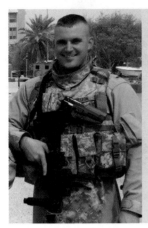

FIRST LIEUTENANT JOSEPH HELTON JR.
September 8, 2009

Photo Credit: Wikipedia.org

Joe succeeded at whatever he put his mind to doing, and always worked to help others achieve their best. He was accepted to attend West Point, but chose to attend the Air Force Academy and graduated in 2007 with honors. After receiving his commission in the Air Force, Joe pursued a career in Security Forces. He was assigned to 6th Security Forces at MacDill Air Force Base and, in November 2008, began training for a duty overseas in Iraq. Joe soon deployed to 732nd Expeditionary Security Forces Squadron as a detachment flight commander. Set to return home in August, he offered to extend his tour and serve with another unit.

On September 8, 2009, First Lieutenant Joseph Helton, 24, went outside the wire for his 44th mission and was killed when an explosively formed projectile struck his Humvee. He is survived by his mother, Jiffy Helton Sarver; his father, Joseph Helton Sr.; and his sisters, Jeanne, Jessica, and Jordanne. In recognition of his sacrifice, Joe was posthumously awarded the Bronze Star with Valor and the Purple Heart.

In response to the outpouring of support their family received, Joe's mother established the Lt. Helton Memorial Foundation in 2010; they are currently working to help fund a veterans' memorial in Walton County and also award scholarships to local students pursuing military careers. The foundations hosts two annual fundraisers: the "Don't Be a Weaksauce" Classic Golf Tournament and the Flat Joe 5k. To make a donation or to sign up for an event, visit www.LTHelton Foundation.org.

HELTON

3 rounds for time:
RUN (800M)
30 DUMBBELL SQUAT CLEANS*
30 BURPEES

Workout Notes
*With 50lbs dumbbells

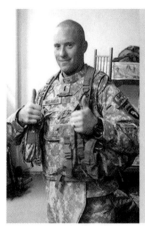

FIRST LIEUTENANT TODD WEAVER
September 9, 2010

Photo Credit: 1lttoddweaver.org

Todd grew up traveling the world, and enlisted in the Army National Guard after graduating high school in 2002. He deployed to Iraq two years later and, on returning home, was accepted into the ROTC program at College of William & Mary. Todd commissioned as an Army infantry officer in 2008 and earned his Ranger tab before reporting to 1st Battalion, 320th Field Artillery Regiment, 2nd Brigade Combat Team, 101st Airborne Division (Air Assault) at Fort Campbell, Kentucky. He soon deployed with the unit to Afghanistan as a platoon leader.

On September 9, 2010, First Lieutenant Todd Weaver, 26, was leading his troops on a patrol in Kandahar when he was mortally wounded by an improvised explosive device. Despite the efforts of his men to get him to medical aid, Todd died of his injuries. He is survived by his widow, Emma; their daughter, Kiley; his parents, Donn and Jeanne; and his siblings, Glenn, Adrianna, and Kristina. Todd was interred at Arlington National Cemetery in Section 60, stone 9183, and was posthumously awarded the Bronze Star and the Purple Heart.

The College of William & Mary endowed the 1LT Todd W. Weaver Study Abroad Scholarship to supports international travel and study; contributions can be made at www.Giving.WM.edu. If you would like to learn more about Todd and his military service, visit www.1LtToddWeaver.org or consider reading, "Losing Todd: A Mother's Journey—Finding Peace in My Heart." The book can be purchased at the College of William and Mary; please call (757) 221-1651 for information.

WEAVER

4 rounds for time:

10 L PULL-UPS

15 PUSH-UPS

15 CHEST-TO-BAR PULL-UPS

15 PUSH-UPS

20 PULL-UPS

15 PUSH-UPS

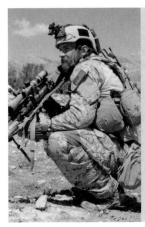

LIEUTENANT BRENDAN LOONEY
September 21, 2010

Photo Credit: Brendanlooneyfoundation.org

Brendan grew up in Owings, Maryland. He spent a year at the Naval Academy Preparatory School in Newport, Rhode Island before accepting an appointment to the United States Naval Academy. After commissioning as an intelligence officer in 2004, Brendan was initially stationed in Korea and later completed a deployment to Iraq. He was then granted a lateral transfer to Special Warfare and started Basic Underwater Demolition/ SEAL training in 2007. That April, Brendan was notified of the death of his close friend, 1LT Travis Manion (see page 68). Brendan still completed the course and his advanced qualifications, ultimately taking orders with SEAL Team THREE. At his wedding reception, he gave his Trident pin to Travis' mother, telling her, "I only got this because of Travis."

On September 21, 2010, Lieutenant Brendan Looney, 29, was conducting his 59th combat mission when the Black Hawk helicopter he was in crashed, killing nine military members on board. Brendan is survived by his widow, Amy; his parents, Kevin and Maureen; his brothers, Stephen and Billy; and his sisters, Bridget, Erin, and Kellie. He was laid to rest next to Travis at Arlington National Cemetery in Section 60, stone 9180, and was posthumously awarded the Bronze Star with Valor.

In honoring the fallen, The Brendan Looney Foundation is committed to helping others reach their greatest potential through educational scholarships, assistance programs, and other initiatives. Please visit them at www.BrendanLooneyFoundation.org.

LOONEY

7 rounds for time:

RUN (400M)

20 OVERHEAD LUNGES (95/65lbs)

[source unknown]

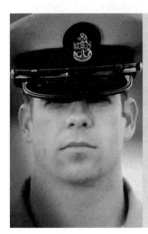

SENIOR CHIEF PETTY OFFICER DAVID BLAKE MCLENDON

September 21, 2010

Photo Credit: Crossfit

David Blake McLendon grew up fishing and playing baseball in Thomasville, Georgia. After graduating high school in 1998, he enlisted in the Navy and trained as a cryptologic technician. Blake was first assigned to Navy Information Operations Command Hawaii, followed by three years aboard the USS Lake Erie (CG-70). He then relocated to Norfolk, Virginia and worked first at the NIOC, then the Center for Information Dominance. Blake successfully screened for a position in Naval Special Warfare and, in 2009, reported to Naval Special Warfare Support Activity TWO in Virginia Beach. The following year, he deployed to Afghanistan.

Senior Chief Petty Officer Blake McLendon was killed on September 21, 2010 when the helicopter he was on board crashed, an incident that took the lives of nine service members. Blake is survived by his widow, Katie; his parents, David and Mary Ann; his sister, Kelly; and his brother, Chris. In recognition of his sacrifice, the Navy posthumously awarded him the Bronze Star.

Before Blake's body was brought home, the residents of Thomasville wanted the McLendon family to know how proud they were of their local hero. The streets were lined with hundreds of American flags, and thousands of people turned out for his funeral procession to pay their respects. Additionally, the Community Foundation of South Georgia maintains the Senior Chief David "Blake" McLendon Scholarship and grants tuition funds to Thomasville County high school students in his honor. To make a contribution, please visit www.CFSGA.net/scholarships.htm.

BLAKE

4 rounds for time:

WALKING LUNGE (100')*

PLATE HELD OVERHEAD

30 BOX JUMPS (24")

20 WALL BALL SHOTS (20lbs)

10 HANDSTAND PUSH-UPS

Workout Notes
*With a 45lbs plate held overhead

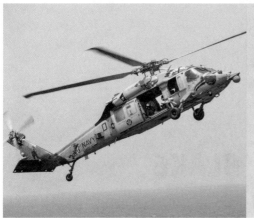

INDIAN 617
September 22, 2013

Photo Credit:
US Navy // sandiegouniontribute.com

Carrier Strike Group Eleven deployed to the Persian Gulf in April 2013. Originally scheduled to return home in September, the battle group was routed to the Red Sea and positioned to take action in response to the chemical weapons threat in Syria. Helicopter Sea Combat Squadron SIX, based at Naval Air Station North Island in San Diego, was one of nine squadrons embarked on strike group's flagship, the USS Nimitz (CVN-68).

On September 22, one of the MH-60S Knighthawks assigned to HSC-6, call sign "Indian 617" was conducting personnel transfers between ships underway and landed on the USS William P. Lawrence (DDG-110) to drop off three passengers. A rogue wave suddenly struck the ship, and the helicopter fell into the water with its two pilots still on board. A massive search effort was coordinated but only debris was recovered. After 26 hours, Lieutenant Commander Landon Jones, 35, and Chief Warrant Officer 3 Jonathan Gibson, 32, were presumed lost at sea.

As their bodies were never recovered, a memorial ceremony was held in San Diego after the strike group returned from deployment.

To make a donation in honor of Landon and Jonathan, please consider Folds of Honor. The organization was started in 2007 to help the children and spouses of military service members killed or injured in the line of duty. As many dependents do not qualify for federal scholarship assistance, Folds of Honor works to provide them with educational support through three programs. Please visit them at www.FoldsOfHonor.org to learn more.

INDIAN 617

In 12 minutes:

RUN (800M)

ROW (1000M)

OR BIKE (2000M)

Then, complete as many rounds as possible:

9 MAN-MAKERS (45/25lbs)

22 BOX JUMPS (24"/20")

13 KB SWINGS (70/53lbs)

Courtesy of CrossFit Coronado
Coronado, California

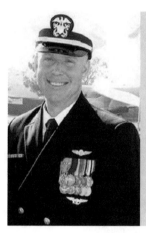

CHIEF WARRANT OFFICER 3 JONATHAN GIBSON

Photo Credit: Oregonlive.com

Jonathan grew up in Kentucky, and graduated from Central Hardin High School in Cecilia. He then moved to Aurora, Oregon to live with his father, an Army veteran, and enlisted in the Navy in 1999. After qualifying as a naval Aircrewman, Jonathan served with helicopter squadrons and completed deployments to Iraq and Afghanistan. He also completed an assignment with Helicopter Maritime Strike Weapons School Pacific, and was recognized as the instructor of the year in 2006.

Jonathan completed his bachelor's degree through the University of Oklahoma and commissioned as a warrant officer in December 2008. He began flight training the following year and qualified as a Naval Aviator in 2011. Driven in his career and meticulous in his work, Jonathan was also a dedicated family man who loved being with his daughter and son; he planned to return to instructor duty after the deployment in order to spend more time at home.

Jonathan is survived by his widow, Christina; their children Makaylin and Alexander; his mother and stepfather, Jo Ann and Mike Lake; his father and stepmother, Scott and Kelly Gibson; and his brother, James.

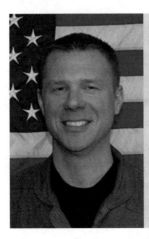

LIEUTENANT COMMANDER LANDON JONES

Photo Credit: Sandiegouniontribune.com // US Navy

Landon grew up in Lompoc, California. He liked to build model planes as a child, and would pretend to fly cardboard boxes with drawn-in control panels. While attending Cabrillo High School, Landon set his sights on becoming a pilot and sought an appointment to the Naval Academy. He was accepted and, in 2001, graduated with his degree in systems engineering. Having commissioned as an Ensign, Landon turned in his imaginary aircraft for a real one: he completed flight training between Pensacola, Florida and Corpus Christi, Texas, and pinned on his gold wings. Landon was later assigned to commands in Japan, Florida, and California, and served overseas in the Middle East. In 2008, he was recognized as Chief of Naval Air Training instructor of the year.

Landon is survived by his widow, Theresa; their sons, Anthony and Hunter; his mother, Debbi; his father, Larry; and his brother, Nolan.

"Our debt to the heroic men and valiant women can never be repaid. They have earned our undying gratitude. America will never forget your sacrifices."

Harry S. Truman

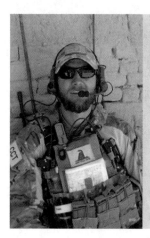

SENIOR AIRMAN MARK FORESTER
September 29, 2010

Photo Credit: Markaforester.com

Mark grew up in Haleyville, Alabama and graduated from the local high school in 1999. He spent two years as a full-time missionary for the Church of Jesus Christ of Latter-day Saints before attending the University of Alabama. Mark earned his degree in finance in 2006, and enlisted in the Air Force the following year. True to his beliefs, Mark never drank or swore; he was a warrior whose commitment to his teammates, his faith, and his country constantly set him apart.

After qualifying as a joint terminal attack controller, Mark was assigned to the 21st Special Tactics Squadron at Pope Field, North Carolina and deployed to Afghanistan with a Green Beret unit. He put himself in harm's way a few months later to direct strikes against the enemy, for which he was awarded the Bronze Star with Valor. Senior Airman Mark Forester, 29, was struck and killed by enemy fire on September 29, 2010 while trying to save another Soldier. He is survived by his parents, Ray and Pat; his sister, Terri; and his brothers, David, Joseph, and Thad. Mark was posthumously decorated with the Silver Star and the Purple Heart, and his call sign, "JAG 28", was retired. Thad Forester is the author of Mark's biography, *My Brother in Arms*.

The Mark Forester Foundation hosts a number of memorial events to honor Mark's memory, and makes donations to veteran support organizations. To make a contribution or to sign up for an event, please visit www.MarkAForester.com.

JAG 28

For time:

RUN (800M)

28 KB SWINGS (2 pood)

28 PULL-UPS*

28 KB CLEAN AND JERKS (2 pood)**

28 PULL-UPS*

RUN (800M)

Workout Notes
*Strict pull-ups
**For each hand

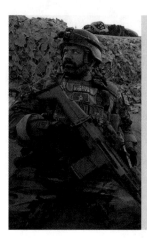

SERGEANT FIRST CLASS AARON HENDERSON

October 2, 2012

Photo Credit: Crossfit

Aaron was raised in the small town of Houlton, Maine. He graduated from Hodgdon High School in 1997 and enlisted in the Army three years later as an administrative specialist. After finishing his first assignment with the 24th Transportation Battalion at Fort Eustis in Virginia, Aaron reported to Camp Zima, Japan. He decided to volunteer for Special Forces in 2005, and earned his Green Beret the following year. While assigned to 5th Special Forces Group (Airborne) at Fort Campbell, Kentucky, Aaron served as a communications chief and, later, as a senior communications sergeant. He deployed multiple times throughout his career to the Middle East in support of Operations Iraqi Freedom and Enduring Freedom.

On September 30, 2012, Sergeant First Class Aaron Henderson, 33, was on patrol in the Helmund province of Afghanistan when his unit was attacked with an improvised explosive device; he was fatally wounded and succumbed to his wounds two days later. Aaron is survived by his mother, Christine; and his brothers, Corey, Sam, and Bob; his father, Dallas, passed away in 2010. On the day of his funeral, flags were flown at half-staff in both Maine and Kentucky, and over 1,200 people gathered to pay their respects at the memorial service. Aaron was posthumously decorated with the Bronze Star and the Purple Heart.

The Aaron Henderson Memorial 5k is held annually in Houlton; proceeds from the race benefit the Wounded Warrior Project. Please visit the "Aaron Henderson Memorial 5k" Facebook page, or go to www.WoundedWarriorProject.org to make a donation directly.

ROCKET

In 30 minutes, as many rounds as possible:

SWIM (50 YARDS)

10 PUSH-UPS

15 SQUATS

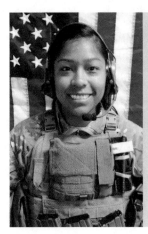

CAPTAIN JENNIFER MORENO
October 6, 2013

Photo Credit: Crossfit

Jenny graduated from San Diego High School, and earned her nursing degree from the University of San Francisco in 2009. She commissioned in the Army Nurse Corps and reported to Madigan Army Medical Center on Joint Base Lewis-McCord, Washington. After serving in a surgical unit, Jenny volunteers the Cultural Support Team program, an assignment that would take her overseas to assist Rangers and other Special Operations units. She deployed in 2013 to the Kandahar province of Afghanistan.

On October 6, Jenny was with Soldiers from the 75th Ranger Battalion on a mission to capture or kill a terrorist leader. They arrived at the enemy compound and chaos ensued series of explosive devices began detonating. Without hesitation, First Lieutenant Jennifer Moreno, 25, ran to the aid of an injured Soldier and triggered the blast which took her life; three other Soldiers were killed that night. Jenny is survived by her mother, Marie; and her siblings, Yaritza, Jearaldy, and Ivan. In recognition of her sacrifice, Jenny was posthumously promoted to the rank of Captain; she was also awarded a number of distinctions, including the Combat Action Badge, the Bronze Star with Valor, and the Purple Heart.

In 2013, the government shutdown delayed the processing and delivery of death benefits to survivors of fallen service members. The veteran aid organization Fisher House offered to help affected families, including Jenny's, to cover funeral arrangements and other immediate expenses. Please consider making a donation in her name at www.FisherHouse.org.

JENNY

In 20 minutes, as many rounds as possible:

20 OVERHEAD SQUATS (45lbs)

20 BACK SQUATS (45lbs)

RUN (400M)

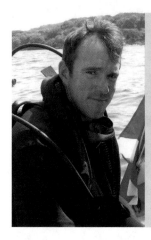

SERGEANT MAJOR JERRY PATTON
October 15, 2008

Photo Credit: Crossfit

Jerry was a native of Bexley, Ohio, and enlisted in the Army in 1989. After earning his Ranger tab, he supported Operation Just Cause and took part in a parachute assault in the Republic of Panama. Jerry transitioned to the Illinois National Guard in 1992, where he earned his Green Beret and was assigned to four Operational Detachment Alphas under 7th Special Forces Group. Jerry completed two deployments in support of Operation Enduring Freedom, and was assigned to United States Special Operations Command when he began preparing for his next deployment to Afghanistan.

On October 15, 2008, Sergeant Major Jerry Patton, 40, was killed during High Altitude High Opening parachute training. He leaves behind his widow, Molly; their sons, Chad, Cody, Chase, and Connor; his mother and stepfather, Cheryl and Stephen Iacono; his father and stepmother, Richard and Joan Patton; his siblings, Scott and Amy; and his step-siblings, Monica, Susan, Trent, James, and Jennifer. Jerry was laid to rest in Arlington National Cemetery in Section 60, stone 8598; he was a highly decorated Soldier, and had earned the Legion of Merit, the Bronze Star, and the Meritorious Service Medal during his military service.

Chad Patton, Jerry's oldest son, was a beneficiary of the Special Operations Warrior Foundation. Through their educational funding, he attended Campbell University and graduated in 2011 with a degree in exercise and sports science. He went on to commission in the Army and served with the 82nd Airborne Division.

<u>JERRY</u>

For time:

RUN (1600M)

ROW (2000M)

RUN (1600M)

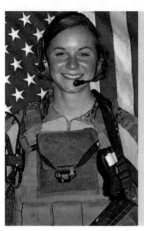

FIRST LIEUTENANT ASHLEY WHITE-STUMPF

October 22, 2011

Photo Credit: Crossfit

Ashley was a native of Alliance, Ohio. She joined the ROTC program at Kent State University in 2005 and, four years later, commissioned as a Medical Service Corps Officer in the Army. Ashley was initially stationed with the 230th Brigade Support Battalion, 30th Heavy Brigade Combat Team in Goldsboro, North Carolina, but was soon selected to join the Army's Cultural Support Teams. At a time when women were not formally allowed in combat, the CST program would get her onto the battlefield alongside Rangers and other Special Operations Soldiers.

During a night raid on October 22, First Lieutenant Ashley White-Stumpf, 24, was hit by the blast of an improvised explosive device and later succumbed to her wounds; the explosion also took the lives of two Army Rangers. She is survived by her husband, Jason; her parents, Robert and Deborah; her brother, Josh; and her twin sister, Brittany. In recognition of her service, Ashley was posthumously decorated with the Bronze Star and the Purple Heart, amongst other medals.

The WhiteHot 5k is now held every year at Kent State to honor Ashley, and the Ashley White-Stumpf Memorial Scholarship is awarded annually at her high school. For information on the event or making a contribution to the scholarship fund, visit www.AshleyWhiteStumpf.com. Please also consider reading *Ashley's War: The Untold True Story of Women Soldiers on the Special Ops Battlefield* Gayle Tzemach Lemmon to learn more about Ashley and the changing role of women in combat.

WHITE

5 rounds for time:

3 ROPE CLIMBS (15')

10 TOES-TO-BAR

21 WALKING LUNGE STEPS*

RUN (400M)

Workout Notes
*With a 45lbs plate held overhead

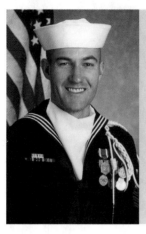

SPECIAL AGENT FORREST LEAMON
October 26, 2009

Photo Credit: Findagrave.com

Forrest was born in Ukiah, California and attended Potter Valley schools until his graduation in 1990. After a year at Mendocino College, he enlisted in the Navy and trained as a cryptologic technician. Forrest completed multiple deployments overseas in Southwest Asia and Bosnia, ultimately earning the rank of Petty Officer First Class during his nine years of service. He took a job with Northrop Grumman after completing his computer science degree, but ultimately chose to pursue a career with the Drug Enforcement Administration. Forrest worked to combat drug trafficking organizations from their El Paso office for several years before joining the Foreign-deployed Advisory and Support Team program.

On October 26, 2009, Special Agent Forrest Leamon, 37, was returning from a counter-narcotics mission in Afghanistan when the helicopter he was on board crashed; the incident took the lives of Forrest, two other DEA agents, and seven U.S. military service members. Forrest is survived by his widow, Ana; his parents, Sue and Richard; and his sisters, Heather and Wai; his son, Luke, was born after his death. He was laid to rest in Arlington National Cemetery in Section 60, stone 9522.

The DEA El Paso Division hosts the Forrest Leamon Memorial Run every October to remember their fallen teammate; visit www.Race AdventuresUnlimited.com for event updates and registration. To make a donation in Forrest's name, please consider the Survivors Benefit Fund, an organization formed to assist the families of those who have given their lives while serving with the DEA. Visit them at www.SurvivorsBenefitFund.org.

FORREST

3 rounds for time:

20 L PULL-UPS

30 TOES-TO-BAR

40 BURPEES

RUN (800M)

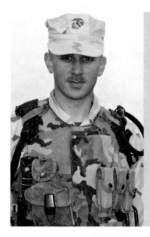

SPECIAL AGENT MICHAEL WESTON

October 26, 2009

Photo Credit: Crossfit

Mike graduated with distinction from Stanford University in 1994, and decided to enlist in the Marine Corps Reserves while attending Harvard Law School. After graduating in 1997 with honors, Mike deployed to Panama as a rifleman with the 25th Marine Regiment, and later served overseas with the unit in Norway and Lithuania. Mike never put too much stock in his Harvard background: when ordered by his leadership to "display his diploma", he complied by affixing his kindergarten diploma to the wall with a combat knife.

While serving on active duty and, later, the reserves, Mike deployed multiple times to Kuwait and Iraq in support of Operation Iraqi Freedom. He joined the Drug Enforcement Agency in 2003, where he used his legal and military experience to target and pursue drug-trafficking organizations. On October 26, 2009, Special Agent Michael Weston, 37, died in a helicopter crash while returning from a counter-narcotics mission in western Afghanistan. He is survived by his widow, Cynthia Tidler; his mother and stepfather, Judy and Steven Zarit; his father and stepmother, Steven and Jude Weston; and his siblings, Thomas, Benjamin, Megan, and Matthew. Mike was laid to rest at Arlington National Cemetery in Section 46, stone 1110.

The Mike Weston Memorial Scholarship was established by Alston & Bird LLC, and is awarded annually to graduating high school seniors in central and southern California; for more information on making a donation, please visit www.Alston.com/ProBono/Community-Service.

<u>WESTON</u>

5 rounds for time:

ROW (1000M)

FARMER'S WALK (200M)*

WAITER WALK RIGHT ARM (50M)*

WAITER WALK LEFT ARM (50M)*

Workout Notes
*With 45lbs dumbbells

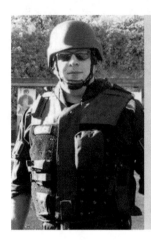

OFFICER TIMOTHY BRENTON
October 31, 2009

Photo Credit: Crossfitoceana.com

Tim enlisted in the Army after graduating from West Seattle High School in 1988. While assigned to the 108th Military Intelligence Battalion in Germany, he ended up in Berlin the night the Wall was torn down; the experience became one of the most remarkable of his military career. He later deployed to the Middle East and served in the Gulf War.

After nine years on active duty, Tim moved to Spokane and began working as a police officer while furthering his education. He joined the Seattle Police Department in 2000, and became a field-training officer known for his dedication, humility, and sense of humor. On the night of October 31, 2009, he was sitting in a patrol car with a student officer when a vehicle pulled up alongside theirs and opened fire. Officer Timothy Brenton, 39, was killed instantly. The assailant, Christopher Montfort, was apprehended a week later and charged with aggravated first-degree murder; he was sentenced to life in prison without parole in 2015. Tim is survived by his widow, Lisa; his children, Kayleigh and Quinn; his parents, Boyd and Penny; and his siblings, Matthew and Betsy.

The book *Keeping a Blue Light On* is a tribute to Timothy and four other police officers murdered in late 2009, as well as the officers who continue to serve the city of Seattle. Proceeds from the sale of the book benefit the Seattle Police Foundation, an organization dedicated to raising support and awareness for the SPD. Contributions can also be made directly at www.SeattlePoliceFoundation.org.

BRENTON

5 rounds for time, with optional 20-lb vest:

BEAR CRAWL (100')

STANDING BROAD JUMP (100')*

Workout Notes
*Do 3 burpees after every 5 broad jumps

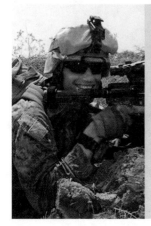

FIRST LIEUTENANT JAMES ZIMMERMAN
November 2, 2010

Photo Credit: Crossfit

James grew up on a farm in Smyrna, Maine and first contacted a Marine Corps recruiter at the age of ten. He enlisted in the Marine Corps Reserve in 2003, and spent a year serving with 1st Battalion, 25th Marine Regiment before accepting an NROTC scholarship at the University of Maine in Orono.

After earning commissioning as an infantry officer in 2008, James was assigned to 2nd Battalion, 6th Marine Regiment, 2nd Marine Division at Camp Lejeune, North Carolina. He deployed to Afghanistan in June 2010 as the commander of 3rd Platoon, Company E. Though his men had spent time setting up safe schools for local children to attend, they were also known for firing more bullets and going on more patrols than any other. On November 2, First Lieutenant James Zimmerman was engaged with the enemy for the third time that day when he was mortally wounded by small arms fire. He is survived by his widow, Lynel Winters; his parents, Tom and Jane; and his siblings, Meghan and Christian. James was laid to rest in Arlington National Cemetery in Section 60, stone 9188, and was posthumously decorated with the Purple Heart.

In 2012, a new Marine Corps Reserve Training Center in Brunswick was constructed and named after James. The University of Maine also hosts the annual Zimmerman Fitness challenge to honor James' memory and raise funds for the First Lieutenant James R. Zimmerman Memorial NROTC Award. To sign up or to make a contribution, please visit their page at www.sites.google.com/site/umainezfc/.

ZIMMERMAN

In 25 minutes, as many rounds as possible:

11 CHEST-TO-BAR PULL-UPS

2 DEADLIFTS (315lbs)

10 HANDSTAND PUSH-UPS

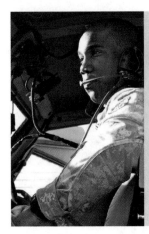

SPECIALIST DAVID HICKMAN
November 14, 2011

Photo Credit: Crossfit

David was raised in Greensboro, North Carolina and enlisted in the Army three years after graduating from Northeast Guilford High School. He qualified as a paratrooper and was assigned to 2nd Battalion, 325th Airborne Infantry Regiment, 2nd Brigade Combat Team, 82nd Airborne Division at Fort Bragg, just 100 miles south of his hometown.

Combat operations in Iraq had already ended when David's unit deployed in May 2011, and they were tasked with maintaining a military presence throughout the area. On November 14, David was in the lead vehicle of his platoon's convoy when an improvised explosive device detonated; he was evacuated from the site with broken ribs, a shattered wrist, lacerations, and brain bleeding. Specialist David Hickman, 23, succumbed to his wounds after arriving at Camp Victory. He is survived by his widow, Calli; his parents, David and Veronica; and his brother, DeVon. David was posthumously decorated with a number of awards, including the Bronze Star, Purple Heart, and Combat Infantryman Badge. As American forces withdrew in 2011, David's death was recorded as the last of an American service member in Iraq. This remained the case until October 2015, when Master Sergeant Joshua Wheeler was killed during a hostage rescue mission in Kirkuk province.

To make a donation in David's memory, please consider the 82nd Airborne Division Association, an organization dedicated to supporting airborne troopers. Please go to www.82ndAirborneAssociation.org/Donate.html to make a contribution.

ZEUS

3 rounds, for time:

30 WALL BALL SHOTS (20lbs)

30 SUMO DEADLIFT HIGH-PULLS (75lbs)

30 BOX JUMPS (20")

30 PUSH PRESSES (75lbs)

ROW (30 CALORIES)

30 PUSH-UPS

10 BACK SQUATS*

Workout Notes
*Lbs equal to body weight

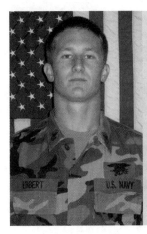

PETTY OFFICER FIRST CLASS KEVIN EBBERT

November 24, 2012

Photo Credit: US Navy // arcataeye.com

Kevin was raised in Arcata, California and earned his degree in Classical Music Composition from UC Santa Cruz in 2003. After the unexpected death of his father, a former Navy SEAL, Kevin decided to enlist in the Navy and initially trained as a hospital corpsman. He then completed the SEAL training pipeline, and reported to SEAL Team FOUR in Virginia Beach in 2008.

Kevin was preparing for his second deployment to Afghanistan in 2012 when he was accepted to medical school at Old Dominion University; he planned to leave military service and pursue his medical degree after returning home in January. While overseas, Kevin spent his free time working in the local clinics, knowing the experience he gained helping the injured and sick would in turn help him become a better physician. On November 24, Petty Officer First Class Kevin Ebbert, 32, was killed during an enemy attack while trying to render aid to other members of his unit. He is survived by his widow, Ursula; his mother and stepfather, Charlie Jordan and Mark Ritz; his sister, Samantha; and his stepsisters, Amy and Kate. For his dedicated service, Kevin was posthumously awarded the Bronze Star with Valor and the Purple Heart.

The Humboldt Area Foundation maintains the Kevin Ebbert Memorial Fund, and makes contributions to organizations that support education, environmental conservation, medical care, wounded warriors, and families of the fallen. To make a donation in Kevin's honor, please go to www.HAFoundation.org/Giving/Make-A-Gift-Today.

KEVIN

3 rounds for time:
32 DEADLIFTS (185lbs)
32 HANGING HIP TOUCHES*
RUNNING FARMER'S CARRY**

Workout Notes
*Alternating arms
**With 15lbs dumbbells

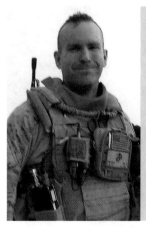

CAPTAIN WARREN FRANK
November 25, 2008

Photo Credit: Crosffitlafayette.com

Warren was raised in Anderson Township of Cincinnati, and earned his political science degree from the Citadel Military College of South Carolina. Upon graduating in 2004, he subsequently commissioned in the Marine Corps as an infantry officer. Warren was initially stationed with 3rd Battalion, 1st Marine Regiment, 1st Marine Division at Camp Pendleton, California and served two deployments in Iraq as a rifle platoon leader.

On November 25, 2008, his unit was working outside Mosul distributing food as part of a humanitarian mission. Captain Frank Warren, 26, was killed when a private in the Iraqi Army serving with their battalion opened fire on American forces; Master Sergeant Anthony Davis was also killed. Warren is survived by his widow, Allison; their daughters, Sophia Lynn and Isabella Grace; his parents, Warren and Rebecca; and his sister, Sara. He was laid to rest at Arlington National Cemetery in Section 60, stone 8745, and posthumously decorated with the Purple Heart.

Warren's family requested that memorial donations be made to one of several organizations, including Toys for Tots. As a Marine Corps charity, Toys for Tots works to distribute toys to less fortunate children throughout the country during the holidays; please visit them at www.ToysForTots.org to make a donation. The Citadel also maintains the Captain Warren A. Frank Memorial Leadership Fund, dedicated to enhancing professional development and leadership training for students. To make a contribution, visit www.Foundation.Citadel.edu.

WAR FRANK

3 rounds for time:

25 MUSCLE-UPS

100 SQUATS

35 GHD SIT-UPS

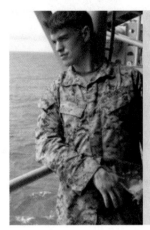

SERGEANT MATTHEW ABBATE
December 2, 2010

Photo Credit: Legacy.com

Matt grew up in California, and graduated high school in 2002. Four years later, he enlisted in the Marine Corps as an infantryman and was stationed at Camp Pendleton, California, with 3rd Battalion, 5th Marine Regiment—the Darkhorse Battalion.

Matt had already served in Iraq and qualified as a sniper before deploying with his unit to Afghanistan in 2010. He was leading his squad on a patrol on October 14 when they were ambushed by insurgents; the team had unknowingly entered a minefield, and several men were wounded by detonations. Matt quickly took charge of the situation: he engaged the enemy, directed fire, coordinated the medical evacuation, cleared a landing zone for the inbound helicopter, and lead a counter-attack against enemy fighters before guiding his Marines safely back to base.

On December 2, Matt's squad was on another patrol when they became pinned down and called in a close airstrike. Sergeant Matthew Abbate, 26, was fatally wounded during the battle and died in the line of duty. He is survived by his widow, Stacie Rigall; his son, Carson; his mother and stepfather, Karen and James Binion; his father and stepmother, Salvatore Abbate and Jane Whitfield; and his siblings, Dominica, Elliot, Valerie, and Kelly. For his actions on October 14, Matt was posthumously awarded the Navy Cross. The city of Laguna Hills officially adopted the Darkhorse Battalion in 2007. Through the city's program, community volunteers provide support to the unit's Marines and their families, deployed and stateside. To make a contribution in Matt's name, please visit www.TeamDarkHorse.org.

ABBATE

For time:
RUN (1600M)
21 CLEAN AND JERKS (155lbs)
RUN (800M)
21 CLEAN AND JERKS (155lbs)
RUN (1600M)

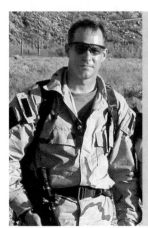

SUPERVISORY SPECIAL AGENT GREGORY RAHOI

December 6, 2006

Photo Credit: Crossfit

Greg was raised in Brookfield, Wisconsin, and attended Marquette University in nearby Milwaukee. He worked for Brookfield's Auxiliary Fire Department as a firefighter and paramedic while earning his degree in criminology and sociology, and graduated with honors in 1989. After earning his law degree from Marquette's Law School, Greg worked as a police officer until joining the Federal Bureau of Investigation in 1997. He later became a member of the Hostage Rescue Team, the Bureau's primary counterterrorism operations unit, and went on to complete three tours of duty in Iraq.

On December 6, 2006, Supervisory Special Agent Gregory Rahoi, 38, was shot during a live-fire tactical training exercise at Fort A.P. Hill in Virginia; he was evacuated to a nearby hospital, but did not survive the wounds. Greg is survived by his fiancée, Paula Paulk; his parents, Natalie and Richard; and his sister, Teri; he was preceded in death by his brother, John. For acts of heroism during his last deployment to Iraq, Greg was posthumously decorated with the FBI Medal of Valor; his family was also presented with a Memorial Star in his honor.

Greg's family requested that memorial donations in his name be made to the Special Olympics: Greg had supported their organization, and took time off work to volunteer and participate in the Torch Run. Founded in 1968, the Special Olympics provides year-round sports training and competition for children and adults with intellectual disabilities. Visit www.SpecialOlympics.org to learn more about making a contribution.

RAHOI

In 12 minutes, as many rounds as possible:

12 BOX JUMPS (24")

6 THRUSTERS (95lbs)

6 BAR-FACING BURPEES

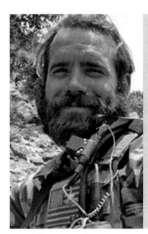

CHIEF PETTY OFFICER MARK CARTER

December 11, 2007

Photo Credit: Honorfallen.us

Mark grew up in the town of Fallbrook, California. After graduating high school in 1998, Mark enlisted in the Navy and left for boot camp that October. He then completed Basic Underwater Demolition/SEAL training and several follow-on courses before reporting to SEAL Team THREE in February 2000. Mark would later serve with SEAL Team SEVEN, followed by the Naval Special Warfare Development Group. During his career, he deployed multiple times to the Middle East in support of Operations Iraqi Freedom and Enduring Freedom.

Mark earned the nickname "Badger" after he won a wrestling match in which, at only 5'5", his tenacity helped him take down a much larger opponent. Mark's otherwise sunny demeanor and dedication to the SEAL ethos earned him a reputation as the man everyone wanted to work alongside.

On December 11, 2007, Chief Petty Officer Mark Carter, 27, was killed during combat operations in Iraq. Due to the nature of his service, few additional details have been disclosed about the mission Mark was supporting or the circumstances surrounding his death. He is survived by his parents, three brothers, and four sisters. In recognition of his sacrifice, Mark was posthumously awarded the Bronze Star with Valor and the Purple Heart; he was laid to rest at Arlington National Cemetery in Section 60, stone 8725.

The Navy SEAL Foundation is dedicated to helping Navy Special Warfare service members and their families through difficult times. Please consider making a donation in Mark's name at www.NavySEALFoundation.org.

BADGER

3 rounds for time:

30 SQUAT CLEANS (95lbs)

30 PULL-UPS

RUN (800M)

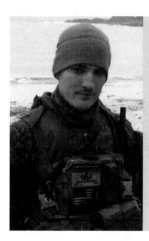

GUNNERY SERGEANT JUSTIN SCHMALSTIEG

December 15, 2010

Photo Credit: Crossfit

Justin grew up in the Stanton Heights neighborhood of Pittsburgh, and graduated high school in 2000. He spent a semester at Penn State before enlisting in the Marine Corps, where he initially trained as a bulk fuel specialist. After serving overseas in Kuwait, Justin was stationed in Okinawa, Japan and was accepted into the Explosive Ordnance Disposal program. He finished the demanding training required to become an EOD technician and completed two deployments in the Middle East.

In 2008, Justin received orders to Camp Pendleton in California to serve with the 1st Explosive Ordnance Disposal Company, 7th Engineer Support Battalion, 1st Marine Logistics Group. He deployed twice more, first to Iraq in February 2009 and then to the Helmand province of Afghanistan in September 2010. During a night mission, Justin's unit was in danger of being ambushed—it was his job to clear the way back to base. Staff Sergeant Justin Schmalstieg, 28, gave his life on December 15 while working to render safe an improvised explosive device. He is survived by his widow, Ann Schneider; his parents, John and Deborah Gilkey; and his brother, John Gilkey Jr. For his service and sacrifice, Justin was posthumously decorated with the Purple Heart and promoted to the rank of Gunnery Sergeant.

The EOD Warrior Foundation is dedicated to supporting EOD service members and their families through a number of assistance programs. Please consider making a donation in Justin's name at www.EODWarrior Foundation.org/Memorial/Warrior/Justin-E-Schmalstieg.

SCHMALLS

For time:

RUN (800M)

Then 2 rounds:

50 BURPEES

40 PULL-UPS

30 ONE-LEGGED SQUATS

20 KB SWINGS (1.5 pood)

10 HANDSTAND PUSH-UPS

RUN (800M)

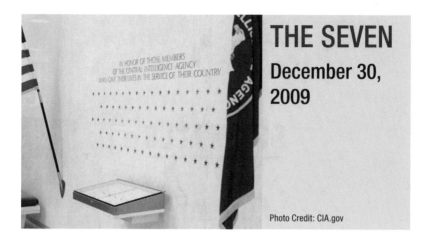

THE SEVEN
December 30, 2009

Photo Credit: CIA.gov

Forward Operating Base Chapman sits near the Pakistani border in the Khost province of Afghanistan. The camp's namesake, Sergeant First Class Nathan Chapman, was the first U.S. Soldier killed in combat during the war. In 2009, a cell of Central Intelligence Agency officers were stationed at Khost hunting al-Qaeda leaders; they had found a man named Humam Khalil al-Balawi, a Jordanian doctor who claimed he could provide information on Ayman Al-Zawahiri, Osama Bin Laden's right-hand man. The possibility of taking out their objective was too much to ignore, and plans to meet with Balawi began in earnest.

On December 30, Balawi was driven to the base for a debriefing with several CIA officers. There were concerns that searching him upon his arrival would cause offense, and security protocols were forgone. When he arrived, Balawi exited the vehicle, cried to Allah, and detonated a vest laden with C-4 and shrapnel. He took the lives of five CIA agents and two security contractors, and injured many more.

On February 5, 2010, Leon Panetta, then director of the CIA, and President Obama spoke at a memorial tribute for the seven fallen patriots. They were each awarded the CIA's Exceptional Service Medal and, in June, seven stars were added to the CIA's Memorial Wall. Because their secret covers had been lifted, the names of the dead operatives were also inscribed in the Book of Honor.

The Triple Agent by Joby Warrick provides an investigative look at the events leading up to the Khost bombing, and profiles the seven men and women killed in the attack. The incident also inspired parts of the major motion picture *Zero Dark Thirty*, released in 2012.

To make a donation in their memory, please consider the CIA Officers Memorial Foundation; their organization supports survivors and dependents of CIA officers killed in the line of duty by providing immediate financial aid and long-term education assistance. Visit their website at www.CIAMemorialFoundation.org.

THE SEVEN

7 rounds for time:

7 HANDSTAND PUSH-UPS

7 THRUSTERS (135lbs)

7 KNEES-TO-ELBOWS

7 DEADLIFTS (245lbs)

7 BURPEES

7 KB SWINGS (2 pood)

7 PULL-UPS

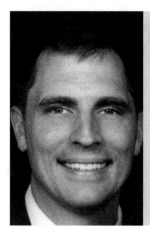

HAROLD BROWN JR.

Photo Credit: AP // nytimes.com

Originally from Bolton, Massachusetts, Harold graduated from Nashoba Regional High School in 1990. He earned his associates degree from Mount Wachusett Community College, and then moved to Washington, D.C. to complete his political science degree at George Washington University. Harold completed his MBA and chose to join the Army, where he began his intelligence career; he later transferred to the U.S. Army Reserve and ultimately attained the rank of major. During his service, Harold served in Bosnia and Iraq, and supported operations in the Gulf War.

After transitioning to the private sector and working abroad, Harold moved to Virginia and began his employment with the Central Intelligence Agency. Harold genuinely wanted to make the world a better place: while working overseas, he had distributed clothing to children and their families, and collected supplies for a local school. At home, Harold was a devoted father and husband who loved spending time with his family; he was also an avid runner, enjoyed camping, and held membership with the Knights of Columbus.

In April 2009, Harold Brown Jr., 37, left his home in Virginia for a one-year assignment in Khost; he was killed by the suicide bomber's attack on December 30. He is survived by his widow, Janet; their children, Paul, Magdalena, and Claire; his parents, Harold Sr. and Barbara; and his sisters, Regina and Paula. To honor Harold's memory, a bridge on Interstate 495 in his hometown was dedicated as the Harold Brown Jr. Memorial Bridge in 2011.

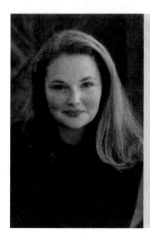

ELIZABETH HANSON

Photo Credit: Colby.edu

Elizabeth was a native of Rockford, Illinois and graduated from Keith Country Day School in 1997. Known for her bubbly and outgoing personality, she loved playing tennis and was a member of the Junior Engineering Technical Society. At Colby College in Maine, Elizabeth majored in economics with a concentration in financial markets and minored in Russian language and literature. She began her career with the Central Intelligence Agency in 2006 and quickly built a reputation for her analytical prowess. Elizabeth had a profound intellectual curiosity and soon became a member of an elite targeting team; tasked with hunting down high-level al-Qaeda leaders, Elizabeth was always relentless in her pursuit of an objective. She was eager for fieldwork and volunteered for an assignment in Afghanistan. In August 2009, Elizabeth was sent to Kabul; she primarily worked at the U.S. Embassy, but the arrival of al-Balawi took her to the remote base in Khost.

After the blast, Elizabeth Hanson, 30, moved to help another victim of the attack when she suddenly collapsed—she did not survive her wounds. Elizabeth was laid to rest at Arlington National Cemetery, Section 60, stone 8978. She is survived by her father, Duane Jr.; and her brother, Duane III; her mother, also named Elizabeth, has since passed away.

Knowing how highly she valued her education, Elizabeth's friends established the Elizabeth C. Hanson Scholarship fund after her death. To make a contribution in her honor, please visit www.Colby.edu/ Memorial Gifts.

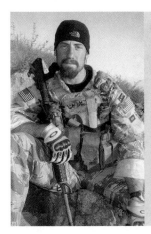

DARREN LABONTE

Photo Credit: AP // washingtontimes.com

Darren was raised in Connecticut and attended Brookfield High School. After graduating in 1992, he walked away from an opportunity to play baseball with the Cleveland Indians, choosing instead to enlist in the Army to become a Ranger. Darren was assigned to 1st Battalion, 75th Ranger Regimen and served eight years before leaving active duty in 2000. The terrorist attacks of September 11, 2001 influenced him to begin a career in law enforcement; Darren first worked as a police officer, then as a U.S. Marshall, while completing his bachelor's and graduate degrees.

Before he was recruited by the Central Intelligence Agency, Darren also worked as an agent for the Federal Bureau of Investigation. He won leadership and shooting awards at the Academy in Quantico, Virginia, and was assigned to the New York field office. Darren resigned his position with the FBI in late 2006 and relocated to the Washington, D.C. area to begin working with the CIA. His job took him overseas to Iraq, Afghanistan, and Jordan; he returned to Afghanistan in December 2009 for duty in Khost.

Prior to the meeting with al-Balawi, Darren expressed his concerns with the security situation: they didn't know the potential informant well enough, and too many personnel were being put at risk. His reservations were well-founded; Darren LaBonte, 35, was killed in the attack. He is survived by his widow, Rachael; their daughter, Raina; his parents, Camile and David; and his brothers, David and Dylan. Darren was laid to rest at Arlington National Cemetery in Section 40, stone 96.

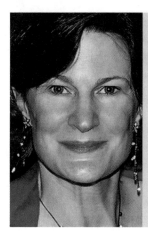

JENNIFER MATTHEWS

Photo Credit: Cedars.cedarville.edu

Jennifer was a graduate of Cedarville University, a small Christian college in Ohio. As a student, she was dedicated in her faith but enjoyed arguing both theology and politics. Jennifer completed her degrees in broadcast journalism and political science in 1986, and married her fiancé the following year. They moved to the Washington, D.C. area and, in 1989, Jennifer was hired by the Central Intelligence Agency as an analyst. By the mid-1990s, she had been assigned to a special unit focused on al-Qaeda and was targeting Osama Bin Laden long before most people knew his name. Jennifer's competence as an analyst and her devotion to her work set her apart, and the attacks of 9/11 only spurred her onward. She often worked closely with interrogators, and managed an operation to capture a high-value terrorist in 2002.

Jennifer spent four years in London as the chief counter-terrorism liaison to British intelligence services; in 2006, she had a role in deterring a major al-Qaeda plot to bomb airliners bound for the United States. Jennifer then applied to become the base chief at Camp Chapman, a job she knew would help her gain operational experience. She received the one-year assignment and left for Afghanistan that September.

Jennifer Matthews, 45, was badly wounded in the attack and died during the flight to a hospital. She leaves behind her husband, Gary; their three children; and her parents, Bill and Lois. Jennifer was interred at Arlington National Cemetery in Section 59, stone 3751.

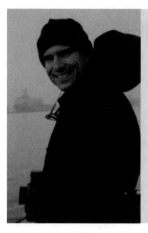

DANE PARESI

Photo Credit: Iraqwarheroes.org

Dane was brought up in Portland, Oregon. The son of a Vietnam veteran, he began Army basic training just two days after graduating high school in 1982. Dane later attended Special Forces training and went on to work as a Green Beret with 3rd Special Forces Group (Airborne) at Fort Bragg, North Carolina and 1st Special Forces Group (Airborne) at Fort Lewis, Washington. During his military career, he completed numerous deployments to the Middle East, Africa, and Southeast Asia, and became a recipient of the Bronze Star. Dane served 26 years on active duty, and retired in 2008 at the rank of master sergeant. He then began a second career as a security contractor and left for an assignment to Afghanistan in 2009.

Known for his dedication to duty, Dane also had a tremendous sense of humor and the innate ability to motivate those around him. He was a family man who had a great enthusiasm for life, and enjoyed fishing, camping, and smoking cigars.

Dane was concerned about the risks posed by the impending meeting at Camp Chapman. On December 30, he accompanied Scott Roberson to greet al-Balawi and quickly moved to confront the informant when he refused to show his hands. Dane Paresi, 46, was killed by the ensuing detonation; his actions that day prevented additional loss of life at the expense of his own. Dane is survived by his widow, MindyLou; his daughters, Santina and Alexandra; his parents, Charles and Janet; and his siblings, Kirk, Mark, Santina, Steve, and Terry.

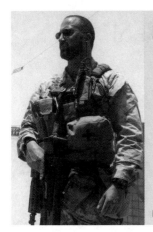

SCOTT ROBERSON

Photo Credit: Charitysmith.org

Scott spent much of his youth in Tolland, Connecticut, but graduated from Sycamore High School near Cincinnati in 1988. After earning his degree in criminology from Florida State University, Scott became a police officer in Atlanta and attained the rank of detective while working undercover in narcotics. He also helped establish the Metro Atlanta Police Emerald Society, a fraternal order that celebrates Gaelic heritage, and loved riding motorcycles with the Iron Pigs Motorcycle Club.

Scott later joined the United Nations security forces; his job took him first to Kosovo, then to Iraq, where he provided protection to high-risk officials. He completed several assignments overseas before taking a position with the Central Intelligence Agency. At the end of 2009, Scott deployed to Afghanistan to serve as a security officer at Camp Chapman.

On the day of the meet, Scott went with Dane Paresi and Jeremy Wise to greet al-Balawi; he knew something was wrong when the man refused to exit on the near side of the vehicle. Scott Roberson, 39, was killed in the bombing. He is survived by his widow, Molly; his parents, Harry and Sally; and his sister, Amy. Scott's daughter, Piper, was born after his death.

The Scott M. Roberson Fund was started by Scott's family to provide financial assistance to students at Tolland High School who are seeking higher education and have demonstrated a strong commitment to community service; the first memorial scholarship will be awarded in 2016. Please visit www.CharitySmith.org/Memorial-Funds/Scott-Roberson-Memorial-Fund to make a donation in Scott's honor.

JEREMY WISE

Jeremy was working as a security contractor when the attack at Camp Chapman occurred; to see the workout dedicated to him and to read his biography, please see page 262.

to see the workout dedicated to him and to read his biography, please see page 262.

"You cannot legislate the evil out of this world gentlemen…in the end, you have to give good men guns and set them loose."

Author unknown

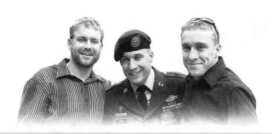

THREE WISE MEN
December 30, 2009, January 15, 2012

The Wise home was a warm one, if not a little chaotic. Jean, a doctor and father of four, taught his children how to hunt and fish, and his wife, Mary, assured they were raised with a steadfast faith in God. The youngest Wise son, Matthew "Beau", learned to play drums and the other siblings played guitar for church worship. G.I. Joes could be found on battlefields scattered throughout the house.

Jeremy was the oldest of the four Wise children; he told bedtime stories to Ben and Heather, and taught Beau how to fire his first rifle. Throughout his life, Jeremy took his role in their lives seriously and sometimes intervened to keep them on the straight and narrow path. He was their protector.

After graduating from West Side Christian High School, Jeremy accepted an appointment to the United States Military Academy at West Point. He finished only one semester, opting to instead earn his undergraduate degree from Hendrix College. Jeremy then began studying for a medical degree at the University of Arkansas.

Ben, three years Jeremy's junior, graduated from the same high school as his older brother and enrolled at Hendrix College. He had once hoped to become an overseas missionary, but floundered in finding his direction and switched to Southern Arkansas University before quitting school entirely. At 23 years old, Ben chose to enlist in the Army and became the first of the Wise brothers to join the military.

Shortly after the terrorist attack of September 11, 2001, Jeremy dropped out of medical school and followed Ben into service. He enlisted in the Navy at the age of 27 and started working to become a SEAL. In 2002, Jeremy washed out of the six month-long Basic Underwater Demolition/SEAL training course that begins the qualification program. He was, in a case of rare exception, granted a second chance. Jeremy finished his advance courses in 2004, and was subsequently assigned to SEAL Team FOUR in Virginia Beach.

Meanwhile, Ben had deployed to Iraq as an infantryman and returned home in late 2004. Jeremy was the next to head overseas, and spent much of 2005 in Iraq. Before leaving for his second tour of duty in the Middle East, Jeremy had met the woman he wanted to marry: he proposed to Dana in 2007, and soon became her husband and stepfather to her son, Ethan.

After graduating high school, Beau had accepted a music scholarship to Southern Arkansas University, but later quit the program. In 2008, at the age of 24, he chose to enlist in the Marine Corps; his mother, simply wanting to protect her youngest, was so angry she didn't speak to him for weeks. The call to military service had now been answered by all three of the Wise brothers.

That same year, Ben completed the Special Forces Qualification Course and was permitted to don the coveted Green Beret. He was assigned to 3rd Battalion, 1st Special Forces Group (Airborne) and deployed again to Iraq, where he would serve as a Special Forces medic. Jeremy followed close behind and returned for his third tour of duty in Iraq at the end of the year. They both came home in early 2009 and, in March, Ben married his fiancée, Traci. He had doted on her two children, Ryan and Kailen, and now they were officially a family.

In September 2009, Jeremy let his service commitment lapse and left active duty. He accepted a position with a security contracting firm, and was sent to the Khost province of Afghanistan before Christmas that year. Beau had departed the month prior for his first deployment, and was serving as a turret gunner in Afghanistan. Back stateside, Ben and Traci were celebrating the birth of Luke, their first child together.

On December 30, 2009, Jeremy was providing security for a meeting between Central Intelligence Agency officers and an informant who they believed to be a valuable source. When the man arrived, he began acting suspiciously; Jeremy and Dane Paresi, another security officer, drew their weapons but were unable to fire on him before he detonated his suicide vest. Jeremy Wise, 35, was killed in the attack that ultimately took the lives of six other men and women. To read more about the Camp Chapman bombing, please see page 252.

Jeremy's body was brought back to the States, and he was laid to rest at Albert G. Horton Jr. Memorial Veterans Cemetery in Virginia. Ben had been sent to Afghanistan shortly after his brother's death, but came home with Beau to serve as pallbearers at the funeral. To recognize Jeremy's sacrifice in support of their mission, the CIA inscribed his name in the Book of Honor and carved a star for him on their Memorial Wall. He was later decorated with the Intelligence Star, the CIA's second-highest award for valor.

Both Ben and Beau went back to Afghanistan to complete their deployments. Jeremy's death had a profound impact on them, especially Ben, who became withdrawn from his wife and their children. He was sent to Afghanistan again in March 2011, and Beau began his second tour of duty a month later. The brothers kept in touch throughout the year; while Beau felt he had found his place in life as a Marine, Ben continued to struggle as he worried for Beau, and missed his family.

At the beginning of 2012, just three weeks out from returning to the States, Ben volunteered for an operation to hunt down a Taliban leader in the Balkh province. His unit began taking fire from fighters holed up in nearby caves, and Ben prepared a Green Beret for MEDEVAC after he was shot in the face. Airstrikes were soon called in to eliminate the threat, but the Afghan commando partner force refused to verify the caves were clear. Ben again volunteered, and pitched a grenade into the entrance before sweeping around the corner with bullets. He was suddenly hit with return gunfire to his torso and legs and, incapacitated, was dragged to safety by Air Force Captain Blake Luttrell.

Ben was given aid in the field and evacuated to Landstuhl Regional Medical Center in Germany. By the time his wife and brother arrived to be with him, Ben's blood had gone septic and his organs were failing. Sergeant First Class Benjamin Wise, 34, succumbed to his wounds on January 15, 2012. Beau accompanied his body home and, in accordance with Ben's final wishes, he was interred next to his older brother. For his dedication to duty, Ben was posthumously decorated with the Silver Star, Purple Heart, and Meritorious Service Medals

Between the years of 2003 and 2012, the Wise brothers collectively served more than 1,600 days in the Middle East, and their family remains one of a very few that have lost two children to the Global War on Terror. Beau was pulled from combat duty after Ben's death, but continues to serve in the Marine Corps.

Nathan Fletcher, cousin to the Wise brothers, started the Three Wise Men Foundation in 2014 to help fight the many issues facing veterans today. Derived from a family nickname for Jeremy, Ben, and Beau, the Three Wise Men Tribute workout is hosted annually aboard the USS Midway Museum in San Diego and at hundreds of gyms across the country. Funds raised through donations and registration support their mission of veteran advocacy; to make a contribution or to sign up for the event, please go to www.ThreeWiseMenTribute.org.

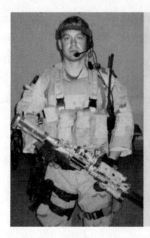

JEREMY WISE
December 30, 2009

Photo Credit: Findagrave.com

JEREMY

In 4 minutes, as many rounds as possible:

5 HANG SQUAT SNATCHES (135/95lbs)

10 BAR-FACING BURPEES

Rest 2 minutes, then continue to the "Ben" workout (page 267).

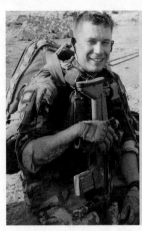

SERGEANT FIRST CLASS BENJAMIN WISE

January 15, 2012

Photo Credit: Washingtonpost.com

BEN

In 4 minutes, as many rounds as possible:

10 POWER CLEANS (135/95lbs)

20 PULL-UPS

Rest 2 minutes, then continue to the "Beau" workout (page 268).

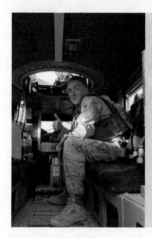

SERGEANT MATTHEW WISE
[Proudly Serving]

Photo Credit: Bendbulletin.com

BEAU

In 4 minutes, as many rounds as possible:

15 BOX JUMP-OVERS (24"/20")

30 WALL BALL SHOTS (20/14lbs)

"Never forget those who were killed.

Never let rest those who killed them."

Colonel George Bristol, USMC

ABOUT THE AUTHOR

A native of Texas, Carter Henry comes from a long line of military service in the Navy and Air Force. She graduated from the University of Texas San Antonio in 2010 and joined the armed forces the following year. Carter has since completed three deployments overseas in support of Operations Enduring Freedom and Inherent Resolve, and continues to proudly serve at her duty station in California.

WORKOUT INDEX

W

War Frank 243
Weaver 211
Weston 233
White 229
Whitten 13
Willy 75

Y

Zembiec 73
Zeus 239
Zimmerman 237